FEASTING ON MAGIC

By The Same Author

Genevieve Davis (real name, Sasha Stephens) has written six books showing how to use magic to transform your life.

Becoming Magic

Doing Magic

Advanced Magic

Becoming Rich

Magic Words and How to Use Them

How to Do Magic That Works

Her memoir, *Becoming Genevieve*, details her personal story and the experiences that led to her discovery of magic.

Feasting on Magic

The Hero's Guide to Ending Diets Forever

Genevieve Davis

Copyright © 2024 by Sasha Stephens

All rights reserved.

No portion of this book may be reproduced in any form without written permission from the publisher or author, except as permitted by international copyright laws.

This publication is designed to provide accurate and authoritative information in regard to the subject matter covered. It is sold with the understanding that neither the author nor the publisher is engaged in rendering legal, medical, or other professional services. While the publisher and author have used their best efforts in preparing this book, they make no representations or warranties with respect to the accuracy or completeness of the contents of this book and specifically disclaim any implied warranties of merchantability or fitness for a particular purpose. No warranty may be created or extended by sales representatives or written sales materials. The advice and strategies contained herein may not be suitable for your situation. You should consult with a professional when appropriate. Neither the publisher nor the author shall be liable for any loss of profit or any other commercial damages, including but not limited to special, incidental, consequential, personal, or other damages.

Book Cover by Michael Warren

First Edition 2024

Contents

First Thoughts	2
1. What's This All About?	3
2. Where Does Magic Come In?	7
3. Why The 'Hero's Guide'?	10
4. How to Make it Work	13
STORY OF A SERIAL DIETER	
5. Let's Begin at the Beginning	19
6. My Personal Call to Adventure	25
7. We've Lost Our Instincts	33
8. But I Have No Intuition!	37
9. Vive La Différence	41
10. Take Responsibility	45
STRAND ONE	
11. The End of Dieting	51
12. The Utter Uselessness of Weight-Loss Diets	55
13. The Life Cycle of A Diet	59
14. Diets Kill Intuition	63

STRAND TWO

15. Practical Tips to Prevent Overeating	77

STRAND THREE

16. Beliefs Create Your World	89
17. Loving Your Body	103

STRAND FOUR

18. You Never Really Lost It	111
19. The Wanting Mechanism	114
20. But What About Physical Addiction?	122
21. The End of Suffering, The Discovery of Happiness, and The Rebirth of Intuition	126
22. Introducing The Hero's Process	130
23. Using The Hero's Process to Discover Intuition About Food	137
24. The Awesomeness of The Hero's Process	149

STRAND FIVE

25. Your Inner Food Guru	155

STRAND SIX

26. How to Deal with Mistakes	169
27. I Get It Right and It's Okay	179
28. I Get It Wrong and It's Still Okay	182

STRAND SEVEN

29. It Only Works if You Do It	187

THE BONUSES

Bonus 1: Superpowering Your Weight Loss With Fasting	197
Bonus 2: Help! I'm Going To Binge!	205
Bonus 3: For Advanced Magicians	214
Feasting On Magic Cheat Sheet	222
WHERE TO GO FROM HERE	226

DISCLAIMER

The information provided in this book is for entertainment purposes only and does not purport to present medical advice. Readers should consult a medical professional or other healthcare provider if they require medical advice, diagnoses or treatment. The author is not liable for risks or issues associated with using or acting upon the information in this book.

I am not a doctor. This is just for fun.

First Thoughts

What's your idea of food freedom?

Are you expecting some fanciful story about being able to eat whatever the hell you like? Some pie-in-the-sky promise that you'll never have to restrict your eating or go on a diet or avoid sugar? If you think magic means being able to eat what you like in whatever quantities you want without worrying about your weight ...

... then you're absolutely right. Because that *is* what magic can do for you and is exactly what this book offers.

Sound intriguing? Then let me take you on a journey. A hero's journey to complete food freedom.

Chapter One

What's This All About?

This is a book I never intended to write.

If you've read any of my previous books, you'll know I used what I call 'magic' to transform my life from miserable, debt-ridden and failing to successful and happy, and losing weight was part of that transformation.

However, since I started working properly with magic, I have actually spent a good portion of this time engaged in extremely unmagical behaviour. Because for losing weight, I *hadn't* used magic—I had used diets.

Magic is about discovering the innate power and wisdom within you and living from that place of truth. It is not about blindly following other people's instructions. So, you could say, going on a diet is the direct antithesis of magic.

Over the years readers have repeatedly asked me to write a book on using magic to lose weight. But I put it off and put it off. Simply because when it came to losing weight, I hadn't used magic.

Until June 2021, that is.

Up until then, I had been on a diet for forty years. Like most people who struggle with their weight, I've been through the usual gamut—calorie counting, WeightWatchers, Slimming World, The F-Plan, South Beach, Jenny Craig, the Cambridge diet, the cabbage soup diet, the Mayo Clinic Diet, Atkins ... you know the story. I had done them all.

It was in June 2021 that I had a revelation that would change everything.

Now, I've become pretty good at making things happen. I've got almost everything I've ever wanted. But I still keep a list of intentions that I would love to manifest or create. Some of them are halfway sensible like 'I want to live in a little castle and keep peacocks.' But others are not so sane, and until recently one goal on my list was to have the ability to eat whatever I want and not gain weight. Pretty crazy, eh?

It was until now. Because I've done it. I've manifested, created or discovered exactly this ability. The epiphany I had in June 2021 led to a completely different way of looking at my body and weight. And by allowing myself, really, truly to eat whatever I want, I lost the excess pounds and am now keeping my weight stable. Ironically enough, it had been *not* letting myself eat whatever I wanted that had led, albeit indirectly, to my gaining weight.

For the first time in my life, I have been able to lose weight without compromising my life, without starving, without calorie counting or weighing food, without cutting food groups out of my diet and most importantly, without the weight piling back on as soon as I became bored.

This story has ended with my losing the easiest, most enjoyable, most effortless pounds I can remember. I am happier with my body and more comfortable in my own skin than at any other time in my life. I feel great, I look great, my skin is clear and glowing, my stomach is calm and settled and my joints feel supple and loose. And unlike any other time I lost weight, this has a feeling of permanency about it.

So how did I do it?

I didn't diet. I didn't restrict what I ate.

I ate whatever I wanted, as much as I wanted yet have lost weight and kept it off. Just to be sure my success wasn't a fluke, in early February 2024, I ran a course called Feasting on Magic with members of my online membership group, *The Academy of Magic*, to test out the ideas. That course was so successful it shocked even me. The members adored it. Many found it life-changing. But perhaps most surprising was how many reported improvements in other areas of their lives, proof that our greatest struggles can be gateways to massive transformation. The book you hold in your hands is the written version of that course. These insights have worked magic for me and my academy members, and chances are they will work for you.

And before I go on, here is a second, somewhat less formal disclaimer:

I'm not a doctor, a dietitian or an eating coach. I haven't done any scientific research, and I don't use academic papers in support of my ideas. To do so would not be in keeping with the philosophy of the book and would conflict with all that I stand for.

You see, this book has come about from paying attention to what appears to be true in my personal experience and the insights I have gained from doing that. I make no claims that you will lose a set amount of weight, and I certainly don't assume to know which particular foods you should eat. Instead, my goal is to empower you to be able to do those things for yourself.

Now obviously, *eating whatever you want, as much as you want* isn't the full story. It's the truth, but it's not *all* the truth. If I gave you that instruction alone, you'd surely put on weight. There is more to it than that. There are things to do, instructions, steps and a plan to follow in this book.

That being said, this plan has nothing to say about eating particular types of food or how much. I will not give you a diet to follow, and there will be no food rules forcing you to eat differently. There will be no eliminating of any food, no counting or weighing. This plan has nothing to do with *what* you eat and everything to do with *how* you eat and how you *think about it*.

Being perfectly honest, the actual instructions aren't even the main point of the book. It will not be sticking religiously to the system or robotically following the steps that will make the magic happen. This plan is designed to give you an *insight*, and your success will depend on the extent to which you 'get' what I'm trying to convey. If you experience chimes of resonance and little aha! moments as you read, if you feel more positive and relaxed around food before you've even finished the book, then this plan will work for you.

Chapter Two

Where Does Magic Come In?

You will have noticed I refer rather often to the idea of magic. But why do I use such an unscientific, fanciful and totally irrational concept? Well, surprisingly, the reason I use the term 'magic' is because it's absolutely the best word for the job.

Over the past two hundred years, we've made astounding advances in scientific knowledge, medicine and technology. Perhaps as a result, in many circles science has become not only the *best* view, it has become the *only* view. If a theory or proposition isn't based on science, it is dismissed by many as nonsense.

However, in worshipping science and rational thought and rejecting everything else as mere woo-woo and superstition, we may be overlooking something of immense value. Some indisputably real aspects of life don't lend themselves to scientific investigation or analysis. I'm not talking about ghosts or auras or past lives but rather intuition, the subjective nature of consciousness, the qualitative feeling of sensation and in-the-moment experience.

These phenomena are crucial to the working of this plan. But despite having immense usefulness and power, they cannot be fully understood through ordinary rational thought. For example, if we try to investigate the subjective nature of our own experience, scientific explanations and objective methods do not get to the heart of the phenomena we are trying to explore. We find that rational thought gets in the way, hindering, not helping, our inquiries.

Sometimes, rather than thinking or rationalising or employing scientific methods, what we need is to stop trying to understand and accept that we can't always think our way to an answer. Instead, we should feel, notice, let go and trust and let our intuition guide us.

And that's where magic comes in.

Magic is the perfect antithesis to rational thought and our frustrated attempts to understand. You can't rationalise it, analyse it or study it with scientific method. It is, by nature, a mystery. But this is not a disadvantage or shortcoming; you can't understand magic because you're not *supposed* to. It's in the mystery that the power lies.

Without the willingness to allow mystery, to allow ourselves to *not* know, to *not* understand, we keep ourselves constrained in our current conceptual frameworks and remain ignorant of any alternatives. When we invite mystery, magic, and *not knowing*, we open ourselves to new insight, new thought and new ways of seeing things.

I'm trying to inspire a fundamental change in you, a paradigm shift. And this sort of profound transformation doesn't seem to come about by taking into account solely the pure scientific facts. It's not that science is wrong or that facts aren't true. It's more that they aren't usually helpful in achieving the sort of understanding we are looking for. So as far as you can, I encourage you to set aside everything you think you know about the subjects of weight, body and food. I'll be honest, some of the ideas I present in this book run counter to everything you thought you knew about diets and weight problems, so you'll need to be extremely open-minded to different ways of looking at things.

I invite you to think about letting a little magic into your life. Don't worry. You won't be required to believe in witchcraft, spirits or energies. In fact, you could be a hard-nosed sceptic and still make this system work. If you recoil at the idea of magic, no worries. Just replace it with a term of your choice or ignore it altogether. The method will still work.

But consider this: On this plan, there will be no deprivation or harsh compromises, no calorie counting and no avoidance of specific foods. You will eat any food you want and as much as you want. Amazingly, you could feel more in control of your eating and your weight than at any other time in your life. I'm not sure if you'd call that magic. But it certainly feels magic to me.

So you don't need to believe in magic for this plan to work, but after a couple of months, it's possible you will.

Chapter Three

Why The 'Hero's Guide'?

This book is subtitled *The Hero's Guide to Ending Diets Forever* because it loosely follows the structure of the hero's journey.

The hero's journey is a near-universal storytelling trope that appears in almost every myth, every fairy tale, every storybook and every film. It was popularised by Joseph Campbell, American author of works on comparative mythology, who explains it thus:

A hero ventures forth from the world of common day into a region of supernatural wonder: fabulous forces are there encountered and a decisive victory is won: the hero comes back from this mysterious adventure with the power to bestow boons on his fellow man. (Campbell, The Hero with a Thousand Faces)

The hero's journey always follows the same basic structure. The story begins with our protagonist living a perfectly unremarkable life with nothing extraordinary happening. Then, at some point, there is a pivotal event—a moment of truth. This is often meeting a stranger or the sudden, unexpected occurrence of a problem or crisis that requires attention. This is the 'call to adventure'. It is an invitation to break away from the mundane and to do something different. The hero can ignore the call to adventure, but the invitation won't expire. It will keep returning, calling over and over until he or she responds.

Answering the call to adventure means stepping out on a brave new path, away from the norm, to travel a less-trodden route.

Eventually comes the key point of the whole journey. Our hero must face and overcome a great opponent, challenge or battle. Having taken the brave step of facing the enemy, the hero receives a reward and returns home a changed person.

We love stories, films and books that feature the hero's journey trope, and those that don't can leave us unsatisfied, irritated or even disturbed because they feel unfinished, broken or 'wrong'. But perhaps the real reason the hero's journey appeals to us, and the reason I love to make use of it in my writing is because it's *real*. The life of every one of us could be said to follow the path of a hero's journey.

In fairy tales, the enemy is frequently depicted as a monster, a witch or a dragon. In real life, the monsters are less tangible but frightening nonetheless. They are our own personal demons and struggles—the things we fear and avoid the most.

In a fairy tale, the reward bestowed on the hero may be literal treasure, gold and jewels, or it may be marriage to the prince or princess. In real life, the rewards can also be financial or some other material gain, but they may also be growth as a person, an increase in status or confidence or resolution of a long-term problem.

But what's heroic about losing weight, especially if we're using magic to do it? As it turns out, quite a lot.

In both fairy tales and real life, the path to success is the same. In order to receive any great reward, to grow, learn or achieve anything worthwhile, we must step outside our comfort zones, doing things that make us quite *un*comfortable. Being a hero may also require going against the crowd, rejecting the status quo or the accepted dogma and opening one's mind to significantly different, pioneering alternative viewpoints. It means not retreating to safety and familiarity, but rather stepping out into unfamiliar territory. To be successful with *Feasting on Magic*, you must take this hero's way. The plan requires you to stop running, face your fears, and go *towards* that which you struggle with.

There is a famous quote attributed to Joseph Campbell: "The cave you fear to enter holds the treasure you seek."

In other words, that which you fear or resist the most is hiding the greatest opportunity for transformation. And through facing those fears, we receive life-changing treasures.

Note also that a hero is not someone who *never* feels fear but one with the courage to face and feel that fear. A hero takes action *despite* fear, *despite* difficulty.

A hero is one willing to do the difficult thing.

So, is this plan going to be difficult, then? Not really. But, I'm definitely not teaching some sort of Harry Potter magic where you wave a wand or do a visualisation, and you're suddenly at your perfect weight. Magic will make everything effortless, eventually. You simply have to make a little effort to get to that effortless place.

Chapter Four

How to Make it Work

There are seven main strands in this book. Each covers a different way of making changes to the way you eat, the way you see your body and the way you view your food. Some will feel more like magic, while others are quite practical. Some may have more of an effect than others, and it's likely that one strand will resonate most with you. But any one of these strands could work wonders.

Each strand contains specific actions, steps to take. These, I call 'magic action steps'.

To give yourself the best chance of making the change you want to see, I recommend you follow all seven strands and complete all the magic action steps. It's important you follow all the steps even if one of them doesn't resonate with you. This is because these steps work in conjunction with each other; in isolation, they don't necessarily have the desired effect. So, if you want great results, do all the magic action steps.

In addition, you should commit to the plan for a minimum of sixty days to give things a chance to settle in and become habit. However, this will be nothing like the diets and healthy-eating schemes you've been on before. There will be no forcing or depriving or battle of wills. These sixty days will not be a hardship;.

Indeed, they *must not* be a hardship.

In order to create lasting change, you need to *prefer* the new way of eating. And I am almost certain you're going to like what I am about to present more than any other dietary strategy you have tried. My intention is that when the sixty days are up, you will prefer this way of eating so much that you aren't remotely tempted to go back to your previous habits.

However, it's not enough to merely like the ideas I present. You can't just read the book and hope for the best. It sounds like the most obvious thing in the world, but you have to follow this plan to make it work.

The process is not particularly difficult. But you will need courage and the willingness to take action doing something radically new. It's this combination—open-mindedness and willingness to act—where true heroism comes in. Heroism is being open to doing something new, scary or unfamiliar and then *doing* it. So read the book. All of it. Follow the magic action steps, and come home with the treasure.

What is that treasure?

Your reward for completing this sixty-day plan is total food freedom. By this, I mean:

- Complete freedom to eat what you want without shame, guilt or fear of putting on weight;

- Complete freedom to eat as much as you want without shame, guilt or fear of putting on weight;

- A greater confidence and respect for your body—being comfortable in your own skin; and

- Effortless weight loss (not guaranteed but extremely likely).

However, as you'll soon discover, this book is about far more than weight, food or body confidence. What I'm about to share with you is almost a blueprint for life itself.

***

What's happening now is that you're hearing the first faint call to adventure. No action is required yet. You need not answer the call at this point. All that's required of you so far is willingness and curiosity. Are you intrigued enough to keep reading? Are you at least willing to consider a leap of faith into the unknown?

If yes, then keep reading.

STORY OF A SERIAL DIETER

Chapter Five

Let's Begin at the Beginning

So here we are, in normal everyday life. Our story has started, but our adventure has not yet begun. We are going about our usual life in the usual way, struggling with weight, doing the usual things to try and fix the problem.

Let's start our story there, shall we? Let's have a good look at this familiar life of ours before we start talking about stepping away from it. I'll give you a little bit of my diet history because I'm sure much of my experience will chime with you. When it comes to weight loss and dieting, I imagine my day-to-day life has been much like yours.

Some of my earliest memories are of my mother being on a diet. In fact, in all her seventy-seven years, I can't remember a time when she wasn't either on a diet or talking about needing to go on one. As a child, I remember our house being full of low-fat and diet products. Horrible stuff such as dried skimmed milk powder that went lumpy in hot drinks, margarines made more of plastic than of food, and a vile saccharin-based sugar substitute called Sucron that made tea taste like rust.

Mind you, Mum was never especially overweight. In the photos from my childhood, she looks mostly around the ten to eleven stone mark (140-154 pounds). (One stone is fourteen pounds to you non-Brits.) Yet she always thought she was obese, and the dieting or talking about dieting was constant.

My own weight problem started early in life. Or, more accurately, my dieting problem started early. I was a tall child who matured early, reaching puberty before ten. This was the age when, for a brief few years, most of the girls were taller than most of the boys. In the final year of primary school, I was the third-tallest child in the school, behind Claire Barrow and Nicola Chase. I was also excruciatingly self-conscious at that age and hated my body. Some children in my class were barely bigger than toddlers. They were tiny elfin creatures, while I was chunky, with breasts bigger than many grown women. I remember feeling big, gauche and bulky, towering over the little cute kiddies in my class like an ogre or a massive lump of fat and flesh.

When the teacher would ask for a 'few strong boys' to come and help move tables or carry boxes. They would include me as some sort of honorary boy because I was big. Being lumped in as one of the boys was all the proof I needed: I was the largest, ugliest, heaviest, buxom lump of awkwardness possible.

The thing is, I wasn't even slightly overweight as a child. But when this self-image of being too big was combined with the influence of a mother obsessed with dieting, the result was inevitable: at the age of ten, I went on my first diet. Yes, ten!

But at age twelve, a miracle happened. I stopped growing. The height of five foot three I am now is how tall I was at twelve. Unfortunately, while my growing stopped, the obsession with my weight didn't. Indeed, that early experience of perceiving myself as too big cued an entire lifetime of dieting. For over forty years, I've been dieting, counting, worrying about weight, controlling what I eat and constantly thinking about food.

Name a diet, and I've done it. I won't list them, because you're probably already familiar with them all.

I've always been pretty good at sticking to a diet. At least, I was good for a month or two. I'd manage this by becoming intentionally obsessed with the new way of eating, buying all the associated gismos, gadgets, the recipe books and overpriced diet bars. I'd chart my progress on graphs and my food intake in journals. I'd also become insufferably preachy about whatever new plan I was following:

This diet is different, don't you know? Haven't you heard? You need to let go of that old dogma. The author of this latest diet is the true expert, and this diet is THE answer. I know what I'm talking about. I've read all about it in this book ...

Basically, I would turn the new diet into a sort of obsessional hobby. But there wasn't a chance any individual diet would become a lifelong change. I'd be pretty successful in sticking to things for around two months, but I could never keep it up past that.

After abandoning a diet, I'd give myself a few days (or weeks) off, to eat whatever I wanted (and often as much as I could). I wasn't a true binger, but I could really pack it away, and between diets, I'd basically eat for England.

Cue the eating-until-it's-hard-to-breathe weekends, the making of a pineapple upside-down cake and eating the whole thing in the space of a day.

But this was fine, I reasoned. Because, thanks to the diet, I'd lost a bit of weight. Plus, I'd been ever so good until then. Didn't I deserve a few days to enjoy myself? Besides, a new diet was starting on Monday!

Once I had broken a particular diet, there was no returning to it. I could never find the motivation to try the same diet twice. The commitment to that way of eating would be gone, and the drive to get back on the horse would be zero. A fresh horse was needed.

I'd heard the old 'diets don't work' advice more times than I could remember. But as I started each new diet, some part of me still believed *this* time would be different.

Any new diet was usually the opposite of the diet I had recently ditched. It would come with a different philosophy and, most tellingly, different *food*. Two months on a calorie-controlled diet and I'd be craving the bacon and egg breakfasts of keto. Then after about a month of keto or low carb, Slimming World green days with their unlimited carbs and vegetables started to look attractive. I sometimes even enjoyed the new diet simply because it was so different from the previous one.

By flitting from one diet to another, I kept my motivation high. I kept my guilt around food in order, and I'd feel like I was getting life right. I felt free and in control ...

...until I didn't. And I would once again give up, stuff my face for a weekend, and begin another diet on Monday.

The danger times came when I ran out of diets. Without a new interesting diet to go to, the weight would pile on rapidly. I'd gain one to two stones almost before I could catch my breath. This convinced me that I *needed* diets. After all, left to my own devices, I was totally out of control. I was sure it was only my constant dieting that was keeping my weight at anything like a healthy level.

And I was never left to my own devices for too long because there was always another diet to try. I'd hear a friend or TV celebrity talking about the latest completely different diet that worked in a brand new way. My ears would prick up, my phone would come out, and I'd have bought the book on Amazon before they'd finished their sentence. That's how it was for forty years.

My discovery of magic had helped me to feel sorted, in control and balanced regarding my relationships, my finances, my career and my place in the world. I was the girl who had it all. I was the woman who could do magic. But when I looked at my weight, my attitude towards food and my history of dieting, I wasn't getting life right at all. What I was doing there didn't resemble magic even slightly. No one could have guessed how dreadfully unhealthy my thinking around food was. And my behaviour was akin to an eating disorder.

Calling this an eating disorder may sound overdramatic. And if eating disorders are defined only by a certain body shape, I didn't have one, because I've never been especially heavy or particularly thin. But if eating disorders are defined by disordered thinking and behaviour around eating, then it's a different story because for forty years, there has been nothing sensible or healthy about my eating.

I mean:

It's perfectly reasonable to think about every single calorie in every single piece of food that enters your mouth, isn't it?

It's perfectly sensible to go on diet after diet after diet, a new one every few months, even though your weight seems to keep creeping up.

It's perfectly okay to deny yourself the food you would love to eat, then eventually give in and binge on it.

It's perfectly acceptable to eat yourself into a sick stupor the weekend before the diet starting on Monday.

It's perfectly rational to label food as 'good' and 'bad' (as if there were some moral virtue attached to them) and to judge ourselves as good or bad when we eat these foods.

It's perfectly normal to fall into remorse and self-recrimination on a regular or even daily basis because of something you ate.

It's perfectly fine that my mother, my sister, my partner, Mike, his mother and almost all my female friends have spent our entire lives either going on a diet, or talking about needing to go on a diet, and spending almost all of this time at various stages of thinking we are overweight.

I want to draw attention to how bizarre, disordered and unnatural this behaviour is. Intelligent, sensible, hardworking women and men, spending forty, fifty, even sixty years worrying about the simple act of putting food into their mouths. What madness is this?

I can't remember a time when I could eat a piece of food without thinking of the fat content, sugar content, carb content, gluten content, animal content or calorie content.

Actually, that's not true.

Most of the time, I was thinking of the fat content, sugar content, carb content, gluten content, animal content or calorie content.

The rest of the time, I would be smothering those thoughts with food, eating to bursting point, as if I could counter those judgements about the food with food itself.

This is no way to live. For me, food had always meant one of two things—weight loss or weight gain. Food was never *just food*. Food was 'diet food', or it was 'stuffing my face food'.

Worry, obsession, guilt, feeling out of control, countered by dieting and restricting, weighing and measuring. This has been daily life for the past forty years.

So, I ask you, is this what you would call ordered eating?

Chapter Six

My Personal Call to Adventure

So how did I discover the answer after a lifetime of such disordered eating?

Like most of us, I put on a bit of weight during 2020. If you remember, that was lockdown year. After six months of home baking and no exercise, I had outgrown nearly every piece of clothing I owned.

I had also become a grandmother, and looking good was secondary next to the business of my general health. I wanted to be a fit, attractive, energetic—but above all—healthy grandma. No problem. I'd lost weight before, dozens of times (even if it has always piled back on again), and I could do it again. So which new diet should I try?

In early 2021, I undertook the one eating plan I had never tried before; I went on a vegan diet. I've been vegetarian lots of times, and for many years at a time. But never had I tried a fully vegan lifestyle. Veganism appealed to me for two main reasons. First, I don't enjoy eating a lot of meat. Second, I have always been concerned about the treatment of factory-farmed animals.

Also, I was inspired by all those Netflix documentaries featuring vegan bodybuilders and those claiming a plant-based diet could solve pretty much every problem known to humanity—everything from curing cancer to saving the planet. So, with a sense of immense satisfaction, in January 2021 I began my vegan diet.

I was pleased to discover how much I enjoyed the plant-based food. Veganism forced me to become more creative with my cooking and to try out a lot of new recipes. I never became one of those evangelical vegans, but I did love the whole idea of veganism and the notion of the new identity—a bit like I had joined a special club. I loved knowing that 'no animals were harmed in the making' of my food. And I was proud to include myself as part of a force for good in the world.

The problem was the vegan diet flat out didn't work for me. Three months in, I felt rotten and exhausted, fuzzy-headed, achy and just kind of *old*. I tried adding extra protein and taking minerals, salts and B12 supplements, but nothing seemed to help how awful I felt. My heart may have loved being a vegan, but my body didn't. Surely, nothing that made me feel that physically bad could be right for my body.

Worst of all, I wasn't losing weight. Four months in I was shocked to find myself at my heaviest ever. Almost without noticing, I had become bigger than ever before.

I gave up on veganism.

So, what diet would come next? Around this time, I read Dr Jason Fung's *The Obesity Code*. In that book, he suggests calories are virtually meaningless. According to Dr Fung, there is only *one* way a person puts on weight. It's not by ingesting too many calories, but only through raised insulin levels. Interesting. *Very* interesting. He recommended a low-carb diet (not so interesting). But that's not all. Dr Fung was also a big advocate of intermittent fasting.

Now, I'd tried a low-carb ketogenic diet before and found it almost impossible to stick to for very long. And besides, I never went back to the same diet twice. An excellent compromise presented itself: The paleo diet, so-called because it is based on what our Palaeolithic ancestors ate, includes meat, fish, vegetables, eggs, seeds, nuts and eggs. But no dairy, no grains, no rice and no beans or pulses. I was sold. In April 2021 I flipped from the (doctor-recommended) vegan diet to its polar opposite, the (also doctor-recommended) paleo diet.

I felt the paleo diet would be low carb enough to prevent raising my insulin too much without the harshness of Atkins or a ketogenic diet. Plus, I had never tried it before, so it provided the essential novelty factor. This would give me enough motivation to carry me through the first few weeks. And for good measure, I decided to skip breakfast every day to create a sixteen-hour fast.

Lowish carb plus intermittent fasting. Restricting not just *what* I ate, but *when* and *how often* I ate. With hope that this would be the answer, I threw myself into the new plan. No diet had worked before, but perhaps *this one* would.

It was odd to be eating meat and fish again every single day. But I have to say, I felt pretty good on the paleo diet. My energy levels were high, and my joints felt loose and comfortable. And the food, well the food was ... okay.

I soon settled into a sort of tolerable boredom with this new regime. I wasn't hungry most of the time, but all the joy had gone out of eating. The food wasn't horrible, but it wasn't exactly yummy either. Still, there was an even greater problem—I wasn't losing weight. A few pounds had come off in the first week, but since then, not an ounce had shifted.

Somewhere along the line, I reasoned that adding in a bit more intermittent fasting might well be the answer. So I started fasting all day, eating only one paleo meal a day at 6 p.m. I lost another pound or two, then plateaued once again.

Keen to find answers, I went to the font of all knowledge, Google, to do a bit of research. After a quick search for 'why am I not losing weight on paleo', I discovered forums full of paleo devotees. From them, I learned that to lose weight on paleo, you can't eat any old fruit or veg. It's often necessary to cut out sweet potatoes and most fruits and go easy on nuts and seeds. So I tried eliminating those foods.

Hooray, I lost another pound. But again, the weight loss stopped.

The paleo diet is supposed to be a lifestyle change, not a short-term exercise for massive weight loss, so these weight plateaus shouldn't really matter in the long run. But there was no way this would ever be a permanent way of life for me. I was never going to eat like that forever. It was too boring, too restrictive, and frankly, not yummy enough. I knew I couldn't stick to eating that dull food and all that sickening meat for long. I had to speed things up, lose some weight and get out.

I suspect this holds true for all of us. The reason we end up Googling 'why am I not losing weight on the XYZ diet' is because we want fast weight loss *now*. We know there's no chance in hell of *any* diet becoming a long-term lifestyle change. We want a diet to provide rapid weight loss so we can give it up and get it over with as quickly as possible. And with the paleo diet, I was absolutely in a rush to get it over with.

After some experimentation, I found that by eating one small chicken thigh with roasted vegetables and nothing but water and one coffee in the morning, the weight began creeping down. Within a couple of weeks, though, the weight loss stalled again. More restriction was needed.

So I started adding in a couple of forty-eight-hour fasts per week, and finally, the weight started coming off at an acceptable rate. Not exactly quick, but by eating four to five small paleo meals per week, I could lose around two pounds.

That's four to five meals *a week!*

But I was far from happy; I was weak and resentful. I'd look at people in coffee shops, average-sized people eating a sandwich *and* cake for lunch and wonder what on earth was wrong with me. I hated that diet. And I knew precisely what was around the corner.

A binge was coming. I could feel it, waiting there on the edge of my consciousness, an almighty self-indulgent binge.

I even knew *when* it was coming.

My partner, Mike, and I had a weekend away planned with friends. A twice-yearly escape to the Suffolk coast with some of our best friends, Sam, Dave and Bertie. Traditionally, these weekends have been four-day festivals of gluttony. The five of us can eat for England, and all of us are superb cooks. Sam is a dab hand with lamb dishes. I cook magnificent savoury pies. And Bertie is famous for, without a doubt, the best roast chicken you have ever tasted. These weekends were a chance to show off our cooking skills, to attempt to kill each other with kindness, and an excuse to eat ourselves a little closer to death.

With two weeks to go before the holiday, there was only one thing for it. I would fast as much as possible, starving myself down to as low a weight as I could so that even after the four-day binge in Suffolk, I wouldn't be too heavy when I got back.

Can you believe this? I am an intelligent, educated, and accomplished businesswoman. My life was a success. But in this one area, I was a spectacular failure, contemplating behaviour so disordered I might as well have lost my mind. When it came to eating, food and weight, I was in chaos.

Fast and binge. Diet and binge. Diet and diet. Diet and binge. Rinse and repeat. For *forty years*. Yet nothing changed. Nothing *ever* changed.

It was on 30th June 2021, ten days before the holiday in Suffolk, that I got up and realised I'd had enough. That was the day it hit me. One of those massive, life-changing aha! moments after which nothing is ever the same again:

I've been here before. Oh God, I've had this insight before.

In going on a diet, I was doing what I had always advised people *not* to do. I was handing over responsibility for my health and weight loss to another, an 'expert'. I was trusting the advice of someone else over my own intuition.

I was following someone else's rules.

How had I not noticed? I was the queen of taking responsibility, of 'changing the world by changing me'. I was an expert in consulting my own wisdom, in trusting my intuition, in seeking answers within myself and never, ever placing the convictions of others above my own. I told my readers and students to believe nothing that didn't resonate deeply, advising them to look only and always to their own personal experience to find the truth.

I taught this stuff!

Yet, in this area of my life, for forty years, I'd been effectively giving away my power to others and letting experts tell me how to eat.

In that flash of understanding, I could see the extent of the problem. You see, it wasn't just that I didn't know how to lose weight. There was something even more worrying: I didn't know what made up a healthy diet.

I wasn't ignorant of healthy-eating advice. Far from it, I was obsessed with healthy eating. For decades, I had kept myself abreast of the latest nutrition findings. From the official guidelines to the faddy diets and celebrity tips, I had heard it and tried it.

The problem was that half the cleverest doctors in the world were shouting some version of 'low carb, grain-free, paleo, lots of meat'. While the other half of the cleverest doctors in the world were shouting 'plant-based' or 'vegan'.

When it came to losing weight, there were plenty of doctors promoting the old calories in-calories out paradigm. Many other authorities said that calories don't matter, that it's the *type* of food that needs to be controlled, not the quantity. Further complicating matters, Dr Fung and others argued that it's not only *what* you eat but also *when* you eat that matters. According to them, fasting for at least sixteen hours of each twenty-four-hour period is crucial. Still others recommended consuming six small meals a day.

So how could I choose a healthy way to lose weight?

Low carb or plant-based?

Calories or insulin?

Regular eating or intermittent fasting?

How could I decide? Which specialist was right? These weren't faddy celebrities we're talking about. These were eminent scientists, doctors, nutritionists. But with so little agreement between them, which one should I trust? There was only one thing for it.

That day, I saw it clearly for the first time ever.

I had to do this myself. I had to stop looking to others. Stop looking to diets. Stop looking to doctors. Stop looking to the latest health fad. Stop trusting the words of others over my own wisdom.

I had to do what I had done before and go back to the truth of my personal experience. The best source of knowledge for weight loss or nutrition was not any specific doctor, study, website, book or diet.

It was time to find out the best way to eat ... *for me*.

Here was *my* call to adventure. My hero's journey was beckoning, inviting me to a fresh way of seeing my entire weight problem.

I knew what I had to do. I knew the direction I had to go. I just had to follow through. Strangely, this path wasn't at all unfamiliar, as I was utterly used to trusting my own wisdom and intuition. But never before had I even thought about trusting myself with *eating*.

Chapter Seven

We've Lost Our Instincts

Have you ever stopped to think how odd it is that we let other people tell us how to eat? Why do we rely on experts for diet advice? We consult them about what to eat, how much to eat, and when. Doesn't it strike you as weird that we need a professional to guide us in something as basic and fundamental as eating?

- *Well, doctors train in these things. Obviously, doctors know more about nutrition than we do! How would I know what comprises a healthy diet?*

But *why* don't you know? Think about this for a moment. You don't see fat sharks or fat butterflies. Alligators don't watch their macros or count their calories. Chimpanzees and gorillas can choose the correct food without consulting a doctor. In fact, no other animal on earth needs to be told how or what to eat. Don't you find that a little strange that humans do? I mean, we're not talking about performing brain surgery on ourselves or fitting a pacemaker. We're talking about *eating*, the most basic function of all living things.

Where does this notion of 'going on a diet' even come from? For three hundred thousand-odd years of human history there were no nutritionists, no dieticians. Somewhere along the line, we forgot how to take care of this most essential activity without professional guidance.

And it's not just with food that this has happened.

We also let so-called experts tell us how to think and feel, deciding which emotions are acceptable and which aren't. Sad or slow thoughts mean you're depressed. Fearful thoughts mean you have anxiety. Bad memories mean you have PTSD. Repetitive thoughts mean you have OCD. Different thoughts mean you have autism or ADHD.

There are even official guidelines on how to sleep (eight hours a night), how to drink water (after or before a meal, not during) and how to wipe our bottoms (front to back, never back to front)!

Let this sink in for a moment.

If you live according to these externally imposed yardsticks, this assumes ...

... you aren't capable of doing these things without guidance.

... you are getting things wrong, and you need experts to guide you.

... there is a normal, 'right' way to be, and you're not it.

The implication is you aren't normal. You aren't right. Your basic functioning is somehow damaged, and you are totally incapable of getting it right on your own. That's why you need expert advice. We are told how to think, how to speak, how to sleep, and how to eat because, heaven knows, we couldn't possibly be trusted to work these things out for ourselves!

But there's something amiss here. I mean, how could you get these basic life functions wrong? How would that even work? How could that even work?

Are human beings so defective that they need outside advice on these basic aspects of life?

I'm convinced it's a lie. All of it.

***

YOUR CALL TO ADVENTURE

So here is *your* call to adventure, loud and clear. Your own journey now beckons.

You are being asked to open yourself up to something new, something that goes against the grain and something you may find difficult to accept. It's this:

> You are not broken, and you never were, but you've bought into a story that said there was something wrong with you. You don't need someone else to tell you how to live your life. You always had the wisdom and the ability to run your life brilliantly. You don't need to be told how to eat, because you have always had the ability to eat perfectly healthily and in the right amounts. You just forgot because you let someone else convince you they knew better.

Now you've heard the call to adventure. So, what's your response? Are you ready to answer the call? Will you accept the challenge of trusting yourself over third-party experts? Quite possibly, you're still not convinced. That's fine. On any hero's journey the call to adventure is often refused at first. But I suspect I know why you're likely to refuse the call, at least initially.

Let's look at that now.

Chapter Eight

But I Have No Intuition!

The reason you're likely to refuse the call to adventure is because you're convinced you have no intuition. You maybe overeat on a regular basis without knowing why. You still need professional help because you have literally no idea how to control your appetite, what to eat to lose weight, how much to eat or what's healthy.

We all started out with a natural ability to eat right. We had an instinct to eat the right things at the right time in the right quantities. But somehow, we've totally lost that childhood intuition about food. Many of us don't know what's best for our bodies or how to eat healthily. We may not even know how much is enough. As I see it, there are three key factors that contribute to almost all problems with overeating and weight.

OVEREATING FACTOR 1: WE'VE LOST OUR INTUITION ABOUT FOOD

How did this happen?

I want you to ponder the possibility that the problem only began when we started listening to other people. In the beginning, this might have been as simple and innocent as watching our mothers control their food intake, hearing them say 'I need to go on a diet.' Or perhaps our aunties told us we had too much puppy fat and should lay off the sweets. Maybe we were told that 'low fat is best' or that 'you should never go to school on an empty stomach'. We may have heard you should only eat 'cheese the size of a matchbox' or 'potatoes the size of your fist'.

What do you think happens when we hear a message (especially from someone we trust) that some foods are bad for us, that we must eat in a certain way or only in precise amounts? We start doing something genuinely destructive.

We begin altering the way we eat.

We might tell ourselves we must fight our desires for the foods we like best and perhaps start believing what we want to eat is bad for us or even somehow sinful. And if we eat the 'wrong food' or 'too much' we feel guilty.

And it's not just doctors and parents dishing out the food advice. We allow celebrities, airbrushed supermodels and low-fat, low-sugar labels to influence what we eat and how we think. It's no wonder we're confused. Our instincts about food and our natural preferences are continually overridden, suppressed, ridiculed or dismissed. Again and again, we are discouraged from trusting our own instincts and advised to follow expert advice instead.

The problem is even if the guidance is delivered by the most reputable and trustworthy source, it has the same insidious consequence: through repeatedly ignoring and overruling our instincts, we eventually come to lose them. We end up trusting anyone other than ourselves, believing that if we let our bodies do what they wanted, without diet rules and nutritional restrictions, we'd do nothing but eat cake and chips all day, get sick and die.

By the way, I'm not down on doctors, and I'm categorically *not* suggesting you ignore all medical advice. A few members of my family wouldn't be alive today were it not for the genius, the compassion, and the quick and intelligent actions of doctors and other medical professionals. So, this book is *absolutely not* a recommendation to stop your medication, turn a blind eye to symptoms and ignore your doctor's advice. I'm only remarking that after 3.5 billion years of life on earth and three hundred thousand years of human history, the idea that we need a doctor to tell us how to eat, well, it's absurd.

Once again, this isn't rocket science we are talking about; it's *eating*, and all I'm suggesting is that you trust yourself to make the right decisions with this most fundamental human function.

Imagine if experts were instead telling us how to *walk* correctly. Debates might rage over whether to walk heels down first or toes first like a gymnast. I'm sure some would recommend walking with your toes out, while others would promote toes in. Perhaps someone would discover a new, better way of walking on tippy-toes, or hopping from one foot to the other. Eventually, someone would come along and say we've been altogether wrong in focussing on the lower half of the body. Legs and feet don't matter at all, they would claim, as long as you swing your arms appropriately while you walk.

What would happen to your ability to walk if you began overriding your instincts and instead took steps to walk 'correctly' like the doctors and celebrities tell you? Can you see how ridiculous this would be? With all that confusing and conflicting advice, you'd forget that perfect, innate ability to walk you discovered as a toddler. In fact, you'd likely end up with an aching back, tense muscles an eventually, a walking problem!

This sounds like a joke. But this isn't so different from what happens when we follow third-party advice on eating. By getting doctors and dieticians involved in what we eat, we're talking about the *medicalisation* of ordinary, innate human behaviour. As a result of this intervention, we've developed learned helplessness with this most basic function.

I mean, we don't know what food is best for our bodies. We don't know how to maintain a healthy weight. Some of us don't even know when we're hungry or full.

We've literally forgotten how to eat.

This is a tragedy and a scandal! We have entire nations of intelligent people who don't know how to eat without outside help. No wonder there's an obesity epidemic.

Chapter Nine

Vive La Différence

Maybe you're not convinced by what I've said so far. You aren't prepared to give up reliance on third-party diet advice. Perhaps you firmly believe we *must* consult doctors and dieticians if we are to lose weight in a healthy way. I mean, these folks are *professionals*, after all.

So, here's a question: which ones should we listen to?

Which experts? What science? Whose research? It may seem right and obvious that we must look for assistance when making food choices, but are you talking about those who recommended paleo or veganism? The doctors who claim sugar is the devil or the ones who point to saturated fat as the villain? The dieticians who recommend eating fruit in unlimited quantities or the ones telling you to back off from grapes? The fitness enthusiasts who say whole grains are good for your heart or the ones who say we should avoid all grains completely?

Should we follow the doctor-recommended vegan diet, high-fibre diet, paleo or low-carb diet, vegetarian, FODMAP, grain-free, dairy-free, gluten-free or sugar-free diet?

Is saturated fat good or bad for you? Is meat good or bad for you? Are beans good or bad for you? Is dairy good or bad for you? Is red wine good or bad for you? Are artificial sweeteners good or bad for you?

And what makes us put on weight?

Is it calories, pure and simple? A rise in insulin? Processed junk food? All grains or just wheat? All carbs or just refined sugar? Just fat? Not eating the right food for your blood type? Undiagnosed food intolerances? Or is it all down to your gut microbiome?

Almost everyone agrees exercise is good for weight loss. But what sort? Weights or cardio? HIIT training or long and gentle? Heavy weights with low reps or light weights with many reps?

Give me an hour on Google and I'll find you revered experts on both sides of every one of these debates. Doctors, dieticians, bodybuilders, personal trainers, even governments and health authorities with wildly differing opinions and advice.

I agree, it seems crazy—even irresponsible—not to defer to experts about diet, but we cannot do this without knowing which ones to whom we should defer.

There are good reasons for the massive disagreements amongst experts. Think about the various weight-loss programs you have heard of or tried over the years. Calorie counting, low-fat, low-carb, Atkins, new Atkins, the Carbohydrate Addict's Diet, the Hay Diet, the Mediterranean diet, Jenny Craig, Slimming World, WeightWatchers, 'eat less, move more', the mung bean diet, the Shangri-La Diet, the Hibernation Diet, blood type diets …

All these diets have worked for some people, sometimes. That is a fact. They all have their fans, their proponents, their advocates. They all also have their critics and detractors. With any diet, there will always be people who are successful and others who aren't. Some will lose huge amounts of weight on the diet while feeling great, and plenty will feel terrible while not losing an ounce.

Similarly, we all have certain foods that sit better with our bodies, while others cause us to react. There may be foods that make us feel tired and heavy, while others energise us or even lift our mood. Some of us feel good eating bread; some bloat. Some love to eat loads of meat, while others, like me, feel sick and heavy. Loads of people enjoy a walk after a meal, while I can't bear it. (It makes my stomach hurt.) Some get hangovers; some don't. Some drink buckets of coffee without any effect, while I am flying after two cups. Some can't eat spicy food; others live on it. And even many of the most effective medications have only about a 55 percent success rate.

What does this tell you? *We aren't all the same.*

Whether we're talking about weight loss, health, mood, energy, intolerances, reactions to medication or responses to exercise, we aren't all the same. So how could there be one objective, universally healthy diet? How could there be a single ideal way to lose weight? How can there be objective food rules of *any* kind, when chances are they will only be right for a few of us?

If you have a source you trust implicitly for nutritional advice, fantastic. I'm pleased for you.

But if you *don't*, there's only one thing for it. You must stop looking to diets and celebrity health fads and stop trusting others over your own intuition.

Once again, as I've taught in every single course and every single book I've written, you must go back to the truth of your own personal experience. It's time to discover the best way to eat ... for *you*.

On this plan, I'm going to say nothing about nutrition or what you should eat because I'm not an expert on your body.

But *you* are.

In a world where medical professionals don't even agree on whether bread or milk is good for you, why would it make sense to blindly accept the words of anyone else?

It's time to take our lives into our own hands. It's time we became the ultimate arbiters of what foods are right for us and in what quantities, because in a sea of conflicting and confusing messages, there's always one expert you can call upon as the ultimate arbiter of what's right for your body.

You.

Chapter Ten

Take Responsibility

A good-looking man sidled over to me in the smoky nightclub, coming close to whisper in my ear. What silky words of flattery would emerge from his handsome mouth?

'Hold your tummy in, love', he whispered. 'That dress isn't made for curvy girls like you.'

Yes, that honestly happened to me. I was actually told to hold my tummy in by a 'well-meaning' and clearly very wise man in a nightclub. I have also been told how to dress to 'make the best of my figure' by male work colleagues and that stiletto heels would make my legs look thinner.

In light of this, and before we move on to the first official strand of the plan, I feel we should examine something important: whose fault are our weight problems?

Should we blame our weight problems on the influence of a patriarchal society, the fashion industry or food manufacturers?

Perhaps you find it reassuring or comforting to blame these outside forces, and I know that plenty of other writers do this. But you won't hear it from me. If you're expecting a diatribe against the evils of advertisers, a weight-obsessed society or white Western male privilege, find another author. I'll have nothing like that in my books for one fundamental reason—*it won't help you.*

It doesn't much matter how you got here or whose fault you think it is.

All that matters is what you do now.

One of my fundamental teachings has always been that we must take complete responsibility for our own lives. You see, if we blame others, no matter who they are or what they've done, we become victims. And when we become victims, *we give away our power.*

Not only that, when you blame external causes or people for your weight problems, you look outward, away from intuition, away from innate wisdom about food. And you can't forge a channel to your own intuition while you're pointed in the wrong direction.

I encourage you not to blame others for your overweight. Don't blame food advertisements. Don't blame society. Don't blame Deliveroo or Uber Eats. Don't blame the big bad patriarchy. Don't blame your mother for never teaching you how to cook. Don't blame food manufacturers for hiding sugars in packaged food.

I encourage you not even to blame food intolerances, your glands, your genes, a slightly underactive thyroid, menopause or premenstrual issues.

Don't get me wrong; I'm not saying these things don't have an effect. They do. It's quite possible you *do* have a food intolerance, gluten sensitivity or an underactive thyroid. It's possible there are hormones wreaking havoc on your body. You may know one hundred percent that you have a real, physical, biological reason for your weight issues. Your mother may not have taught you to cook, and you may have been bombarded by advertisements depicting skinny women, and you may have been bullied for being fat as a child, and you may feel the oppressive influence of the big bad patriarchy.

These issues are genuine. I'm not denying that. There is not a level playing field when it comes to weight loss. You may well have circumstances that make it more difficult for you to lose weight. Many of us do. But can you get into the habit of taking responsibility even when there are factors at play that make it harder for you?

After all, I've talked at length about the negative effects of conflicting health advice and the big part dieting has played in our problems with weight and eating. My obsession with dieting almost certainly started because of my mother's influence. Society's views on weight have doubtless also had a negative effect on me. I've become confused by experts who disagree on nutrition. I'm also fifty-five and, by most reckoning, should be slap-bang in the middle of menopause. But do I blame these external factors?

Never. Because not one of these negative influences eliminates my responsibility to change things. If we blame the parents, the creators of diets, the food companies, the patriarchy, we end up passing the responsibility to another. And when we do this, even a little, we end up disempowering ourselves.

Please don't misunderstand me. Taking responsibility is not about blaming the victim. It's not about blaming *anyone*. It's about working with the hand you've been dealt, however great or crappy it may be. And it's about not using a slightly poor hand as an excuse to do *nothing*.

Work with what you've got. Do what you can. Because no one is going to do it for you. Even if it is their fault.

***

THE FINAL CALL TO ADVENTURE

So, it's now time to answer your call to adventure. This is your last chance to refuse. You can still turn back at this point. You can retreat into the same old way of doing things.

We are about to start the first strand of the plan. If you're going to continue, you will have to step away from your conventions, away from what you thought was true, away from the old life to embrace these new possibilities.

It's time to take responsibility, defy conventions, break away from the norm. To try something radically different and embark on a bold and uncharted voyage. To take action despite all those around you telling you to do otherwise. We are now leaving the everyday world. From this point on, life will never be the same.

Ready? Then let's step out on your hero's journey to food freedom.

STRAND ONE

NO RESTRICTIONS, NO RULES, NO DIETS

Chapter Eleven

The End of Dieting

One big promise I make in this book is that you will be able to turn your back on diets for good. So I'm going to start this section by explaining why I'm so down on diets. One thing I will demonstrate is that weight-loss diets are a big factor in keeping you overweight.

You may be convinced that diets are all that's keeping your weight in check and that without these restrictions you'd surely eat yourself to death. This fear is perhaps the number one reason we turn to third parties for diet advice.

I bought into this with all my heart and soul. I genuinely took for granted that if I stopped my constant dieting, I'd be out of control. The evidence appeared to support this. After all, when I dieted, my weight would go down. When I stopped, my weight would go up. As a result, I was convinced only my nearly constant dieting kept me anything close to a healthy weight. If I ever let go of my tight control on food, my calorie counting and my yo-yo dieting, surely I would become morbidly obese.

In two to five years, I would resemble Jabba the Hutt (so I imagined). And, having eaten myself literally to death, my lifeless body would be dragged out of my house on a tarpaulin after firefighters had smashed a hole in the wall to get me out.

It was only diets that prevented this nightmare. I was sure of it. Hence for forty years I have been:

1. on a diet;

2. looking to go on a diet; or

3. finishing up a diet (and preparing to start another one).

Do you know the seriously tragic thing? It hasn't worked. With each passing decade, my weight has gone up a stone. In my teens I was seven-stone-something, in my twenties, it was eight-stone-something, thirties were nine-stone-something, forties were ten-stone-something. And as I hit my early fifties, I was eleven stone eleven pounds (165 pounds). That's quite a lot to carry on my little five-foot-three frame. If the pattern continued, my sixties would see me at *well* over twelve stone (168 pounds).

Then last year it finally dawned on me:

Diets have *not* fulfilled their promise. They have not worked as advertised. Diets have not prevented me from becoming overweight. Truth is: *diets don't work*. And I have forty years of experience to prove it.

I know it's hard to accept that without the structure of a diet you would be capable of regulating your own eating. Maybe you even have a similar nightmare to my Jabba-through-the-wall scenario.

But let me ask: How long have you been dieting? Haven't you noticed that it's never worked? Sure, you've lost bits and pieces of weight over the years, but hasn't that weight always gone back on?

- *It's that I haven't found the right diet. If I could just find one I could stick to.*

Seriously?

How many *decades* has it been that you've been trying to lose this weight? Go on, count them up. How many diets have you been on? Six, twenty, a hundred? Haven't you noticed your weight creeping up and up despite all these diets? What makes you think *another* diet is going to be different? That this next one will be the one that works? What makes you think this trend won't continue? After all, despite all these diets, you're still here, reading this book, trying to lose weight.

So, when are you going to catch on? *It's not working.*

It's not working because *diets don't work*. If you carry on going on diet after diet, nothing is ever going to change. Except your weight, that is. Your weight might well increase, as it always has before.

It's no wonder we diet and binge and jump from one weight-loss fad to another. We are trapped in a vicious circle that repeats over and over and over, bouncing around between diets, turning from one set of rules to another, never stopping to question the whole mechanism beneath what we are doing, never realising it's not *us* that are wrong. It's the *dieting* that's wrong. It's not *any particular diet* that's wrong; it's the fact that there's a diet at all. There's a popular saying that insanity is doing the same thing over and over and expecting different results. It's time to stop that insanity.

- But it's not the diets that fail; it's people that fail. Diets do work, it's people that don't do them properly. Diets would work if people had enough willpower to stick to them.

So, this means, *diets* work, but people *don't*. Diets would work if only people were stronger, less useless or flaky, more disciplined, or better educated.

I call bullshit.

Did you know that over 80 percent of people who lose weight on a diet will gain that weight back within a year?

Eighty percent!

How can a diet be considered effective when it doesn't work for 80 percent of people? A medical treatment or medication with an 80 percent failure rate would be banned. You wouldn't blame the 80 percent of people who took that medication because they didn't get better. You wouldn't call them weak, uneducated or undisciplined.

If you have tried and failed with diets, rest assured, this is normal. It's what everyone experiences. The reason diets haven't worked for you is not that you are stupid or greedy, or that you don't have enough willpower to stick to them. Neither is it because you haven't found the right one.

Diets don't work because they *cannot* work.

Chapter Twelve

The Utter Uselessness of Weight-Loss Diets

You've likely heard the phrase 'diets don't work' lots of times. You may have heard that the body goes into starvation mode on a very low-calorie diet, that metabolism slows down. When you stop dieting, your body starts hanging on to fat, and you end up weighing more than before you even started the diet.

This may all be true, but it's not what I'm going to talk about in this book. I've noticed something very different at play that makes *all* restrictive diets hopeless for long-term weight loss.

What I'm talking about appears to have been excluded from the standard dogma around weight gain and loss. It fits into neither the calories-in-calories-out model nor the raised-insulin model. Nonetheless it's something so obvious and intuitively correct it's incredible no one is talking about it.

Diets don't work because the mechanism by which they are supposed to work prevents them from working.

To understand this, it's necessary to explore why we eat. The obvious answer is that the body needs fuel. A signal of hunger tells us it's time to eat when our reserves are running low. In other words, we eat to fuel our bodies and keep them working.

So why do we *overeat*? Many of us regularly eat more than is comfortable. If eating were solely about hunger, overeating wouldn't even be a thing. So 'food is fuel' clearly isn't the full picture.

Is it that we're all greedy and weak-willed?

Far from it.

To understand why we overindulge, we need to appreciate something of vital importance. *Eating is about more than hunger.*

Human beings aren't machines in need of fuel alone. A human being has an emotional side, a spiritual aspect, a *soul* if you like to speak in such terms. And souls need nourishment as much as bodies. This is the reason human beings enjoy music, art, poetry and hobbies. We don't engage in these pastimes for the survival of our physical bodies—we do so to feed our souls. We also need love and friendship and purpose in order to thrive. And we need *food we enjoy.*

Human beings do not consume food only for nutrition or to sate hunger, and we never have. We use food for celebrations, to mark festivals and milestones and to punctuate the year. All cultures do this and have done so for millennia.

Eating is not about mere hunger, but about enjoyment. We eat to create a feeling of fullness, not solely in the stomach, but in a more all-over sense. We eat to provide body and soul satisfaction.

Now, here's where it gets interesting. If we don't get full, all-over, body and soul satisfaction from our food, we tend to keep eating. And we'll do this *even when we are no longer hungry*. When we continue to eat after our nutritional and hunger requirements have been fulfilled, this is always an effort to satisfy the soul. And so, we come to the second of three key factors in overeating.

OVEREATING FACTOR 2: LACK OF SATISFACTION

Truth is, we aren't getting enough satisfaction from our food. But why? Most of us live in societies where food is delicious and plentiful. We can have literally hundreds of exotic foods delivered to our doorsteps at the tap of a button on our phones. What's wrong with us? All this delicious food on offer and we aren't satisfied.

Well, here's the thing—if we are serial dieters, we aren't truly *allowed* all that delicious food, are we? We don't have free rein to enjoy whatever exotic and satisfying food we want. To prove this, think about your answers to these questions

- When you are making a choice about what to eat, do you often make that choice based on whether it is fattening or non-fattening?
- Do you leave the mayonnaise off your sandwich, the cream off your apple pie, or the dressing off your salad to reduce the calories?
- Do you tot up the rough number of calories in a meal before deciding to eat it?
- Do you usually choose the meal you think is likely to be lower in carbs, sugar or fat?
- Do you always choose a meal because it's what you really want?
- Do you usually make eating decisions based mainly on possible effects on your weight?

I propose that selecting food based not on deliciousness but on weight-related concerns has the opposite effect to the one we want. Far from helping us stay slim, forgoing the foods we want in favour of those we believe will keep us slender usually leads to overeating.

This is especially true when you follow a specific weight-loss diet.

Chapter Thirteen

The Life Cycle of A Diet

When you start out on a new weight-loss diet, usually your motivation is high. You make a couple of the recommended diet meals, and the food seems perfectly acceptable. It's not quite what you want, but it's still tasty and your tummy is full enough. You begin to lose weight, and all seems well.

Then comes that point, a couple of weeks into the diet when your soul starts to cry out for satisfaction. This is when you begin to crave yummy foods.

At the beginning of a diet, your willpower is usually strong enough to silence and overrule these urges, but eventually there will be a revolution against the diet. This is when the oh-so-convincing sabotage thoughts begin to pop in.

One bar of chocolate won't hurt. You can be extra good tomorrow. This diet isn't working anyway. That new diet you heard about is going to work far better than this. Go on, have some chocolate, and start again on Monday.

That initial motivation becomes outgunned by other voices that grow louder until your willpower starts to falter. An almighty battle of wills sets in as your body tries to compel you to go off-diet and eat something delicious. Sometimes, your willpower wins out and you stick to the diet. Other times, the voices win out, you break the diet, and you eat the yummy food, *lots* of it.

I want you to realise that when this happens, it is not a lack of will or some sort of character flaw. Just as a lonely person will eventually seek company; a person starved, not of food, but of the *enjoyment* of food, will ultimately rebel against the diet.

Those seemingly traitorous thoughts are not signs of a weak character or lack of control. They are a natural, healthy response. They are warning us something is wrong.

Let's look at how diets are supposed to work. What unites all diets, all diet rules and all weight-management guidelines? Even among such diverse regimes as veganism and the Atkins diet, WeightWatchers and Slimming World, Slimfast, and the Cambridge diet, there is one common feature:

Restriction.

Diets, by necessity, restrict either what you may eat, in what quantities, or both. Whether it's banned foods, limited portions or numbers of calories, diets are, by definition, about restriction.

But there's another word we could use instead of restriction:

Deprivation.

All diets are deprivation plans. Diet rules are necessary because, left to your own devices, you would eat something else. If not, there would be no need for the diet in the first place. Going on a diet then, by definition, means depriving yourself of what, or how much, you want to eat.

It is this very mechanism—restriction, or, more accurately, *deprivation*—that dooms diets to failure. In other words, the fundamental way in which diets function actually stops them working.

Think about it. How often have you finished a diet meal and felt unsatisfied? You might be physically full, but the meal was still somehow lacking. When you take steps to make sure the food on your plate is as low calorie, as low carb or as low fat as possible, it's less delicious than you want it to be. This means the chances of getting full satisfaction are nil.

People on a diet often feel the joy has gone out of eating because the food they consume isn't hitting the mark. Eating a whole loaf of stale bread will fill your tummy, but it isn't likely to leave you satisfied. So even diets that allow you to eat unlimited quantities of some foods don't tend to last long. It doesn't matter how full your stomach is on diet food, as long as you're eating food that doesn't feed your soul or nourish your entire being, you're going to want more. This is what makes it so hard to stick to a diet.

Interestingly, I have a couple of male friends who occasionally go on the mung bean diet. Apparently, mung beans are a perfectly balanced meal in themselves, and my two friends will lose a fair bit of weight by eating nothing else for a few weeks. But even though mung beans are filling and nutritionally almost a complete meal, these chaps still can't stick to the diet for more than a couple of weeks. Why? Because it's boring. It doesn't satisfy the soul. Eating nothing but mung beans leaves them miserable, unsatisfied, and eventually almost desperate for delicious food.

Going on any diet is not so different to the mung bean diet. They differ only in degree. Granted, most diets are far less extreme, but they all have one thing in common—*they don't satisfy*. As a result, when you break a diet, it's hardly ever exclusively about hunger; it's about an overwhelming urge to find satisfaction. Again, if we could get full satisfaction from the food on a diet, there would be no need for the diet rules in the first place—we'd simply eat that food by choice.

So let's stop pretending food is all about hunger. It doesn't matter how full your tummy is on diet food, when you deprive yourself of food that you actually want, part of you is going to yell for something else.

Indeed, when you're on a diet, I suspect the reason you end up craving everything you're not allowed is that your inner wisdom, the intuitive part of you, is trying to make itself heard, and it *knows* the most effective way to make you stop the restriction. It *encourages* you to eat 'bad' things like chocolate or ice cream because that's the fastest way to get you off the diet. So when you break a diet and eat ice cream, it's not some moral failing. You aren't getting it wrong—*you're getting it right!* Your body knows what's good for you. And when it forces you to break a diet, it's telling you that *this diet is not good for you!*

I put it to you that if a diet isn't delicious and satisfying, it's not a healthy diet. And if we aren't nourishing the soul as well as the stomach, we aren't properly feeding at all.

We are vibrant, loving, joyful, magical beings, and we require enjoyment and satisfaction in order to work at our highest level. We need love, we need joy, we need belonging, we need purpose, we need spiritual fulfilment and we need satisfaction from our food. In short: we can't live on mung beans alone!

Chapter Fourteen

Diets Kill Intuition

We began losing our intuition about food when we began letting other people tell us how to eat. For most people reading this book, the most destructive way we have done this is by constantly dieting, going from one third-party set of restrictions to another, silencing and ignoring our natural proclivities to eat the things we enjoy.

Dieting is probably the biggest reason we've lost our intuition. We've been overriding our instincts with diet after diet for so long that our ability to hear our intuition is almost zero. And we can't even contemplate trusting ourselves to manage our weight without outside help.

Diets involve an almost arrogant disregard for your own intelligence, your wisdom and intuition. They mean defying your own natural inclinations, and as a consequence, *by design*, denying you satisfaction.

- *But at least I DO lose weight on a diet.*

This is perhaps the worst part. To add insult to injury, if you *do* manage to lose weight on a diet, you can't even claim that for yourself. After all, it was the *diet* that made you lose all that weight. It was the *diet* that worked, not you. Let's face it, you couldn't possibly have done it on your own!

Going on a diet is thus a quick fix, like taking steroids to make you develop muscles or taking sleeping pills to help you sleep. Yes, these things work in the short term, kind of. But long term they reinforce the idea that you can't do anything worthwhile without outside help.

Your intuition to make the right food choices weakens after every single diet you try, even when you lose weight, further damaging your ability to trust yourself.

Thus, diets kill intuition, even when they appear to work.

And if you break a diet *without* losing weight, you become further demoralised. You've been taught to associate stopping a diet with failure, with giving up, with lack of willpower, with a flawed character and a greedy stomach. It's no wonder hell breaks loose once you're off the diet. Without the false security of the rules, you are left to your own devices, having to be responsible for your own eating and your own weight. But thanks to the diet, you've lost your intuition and have no access to your own perfect wisdom. You're on your own. Lost and out of control.

See why I'm so down on diets?

For decades, you have maintained the idea that dieting is the only way to keep in control of your weight. It's now time to change that.

You are on a hero's journey, a quest to find an incredible capacity that has been hidden, out of sight for such a long time you forgot it was there. Somewhere inside of you is a quiet but perfect intuition about food.

We need to get our hands on that lost treasure.

This inner voice of intuition has the perfect knowledge of *what* to eat, *when* to eat, *how much* to eat, and when to *stop*. It also knows exactly the right food to give us both the perfect nutrition for our bodies, plus the all-over, body and soul satisfaction we crave. It's that voice that we are going to discover during the next sixty days.

MAGIC ACTION STEP: EAT WHAT YOU WANT

It's time to take our first magic action step on this path to a new life. I now introduce the first formal instruction of this plan.

You must eat whatever you want[1].

We put restrictions on what we eat because we don't trust ourselves. When there is no trust, there is a lack of connection to intuition, and it is impossible to make knowingly sound eating choices. In order to access your intuition you must offer yourself the chance to trust yourself, and that's not possible when there are restrictions in place.

The *sole* way to contact that inner, perfect wisdom about food is experimenting with *no* restrictions. *No* diets. *No* food charts. *No* eating guidelines. That means the days of picking the low-fat option, the lower calorie meal, the lower carb choice or the meal you think you *should* eat are over. The way to an intuitive ability to eat the right things in the right amounts is not restriction, not deprivation, *but the lack of them*. It may seem counterintuitive, intimidating, even ridiculous, but this step is essential. You *must* eat whatever you want.

Some years ago, I wrote a book called *Becoming Rich*. In that book, I tell the ever so cool rags-to-riches story of how I transformed my financial situation from poverty and debt to wealth and success. I did this largely by working out a way to think and behave like a rich person *before I was rich*. The money that then came to me was the inevitable consequence of that change in me.

---

1. If you're diabetic or you have a known intolerance or allergy to something, obviously follow expert advice. But if you have no medical reasons not to, you must choose to eat whatever you like given the choices on offer.

When we struggle financially, we usually think about money in a longing, lacking way. We worry and whine about not having enough, and we fantasise about how perfect life would be if only we had more. But the more we hanker after money, the more it gets tied up with notions of power and control, good and bad, regret, shame and blame, fear and loss. All this confused and messy thinking involved in dealing with money, and this constant focus on *lack*, makes it almost impossible for us to get more of it.

In *Becoming Rich*, I teach readers how to become neutral regarding money. When we learn to stop stressing, worrying about and yearning for money, we become relaxed about the whole subject, and we begin acting more like rich people. Money then becomes vastly easier to get.

While I was writing *Feasting on Magic*, I came to realise my stressing around food was almost exactly analogous to worrying and complaining and obsessing about money.

After all, I had nothing *like* a neutral attitude toward food.

Restricting food, planning food, eating food, guilt about eating too much food, cravings, diets, selecting diets, deciding to break diets, disgrace at having broken a diet, dissatisfaction at my body, longing for a slimmer one. These thoughts and actions had dictated my eating almost my entire adulthood. Dieting and calorie control were such dominant forces in my life that I felt incapable of coping without them.

If thinking and acting like a rich person before I was rich had led to my *becoming* rich, perhaps I could do the same thing with my weight. Could I become relaxed and neutral around food before I was thin?

There would be no point in learning from successful dieters; I wanted to emulate people who had *never* been on a diet. I looked at my naturally thinner friends to see how they behaved. I watched slim people in restaurants. What was the difference between them and me? What and how did they eat? How did they behave around this whole subject of food, weight and eating?

- *I suppose all those skinny people live on rice cakes and lettuce. Do they? Or miso soup and celery?*

Far from it. When I looked at my naturally thinner friends, and even at strangers, they were tucking into desserts and potatoes and full-fat mayonnaise. I didn't see them: a) cutting out sugar or b) cutting out fat. I didn't see them counting calories. In fact, the thin people seemed to eat more or less whatever they liked, while I was obsessed with what I should and shouldn't eat, restricting this, cutting out that and counting everything.

Then it hit me: this exact behaviour was part of the problem. After all, what naturally slim person does this? They think, feel and act like thin people. Whereas I was acting, well, kind of like a fat person.

- *But what about all those diets you followed? That wasn't acting like a fat person.*

Yes, it was! This was the worst of it. How many overweight people do you know who have been on multiple diets? Almost every single one of them. In fact, I bet all the overweight people you have ever known have been serial dieters.

Naturally slim people don't go on diets. They don't cut out sugar or fat. They don't count calories. They don't deprive themselves. Naturally thin people eat what they like, when they like, without even thinking about it. They don't obsess and fill their every waking moment with thoughts about food and dieting. They stay slim *because* they don't think about it.

Naturally thin people are relaxed and in control around food. They eat what they like, intuitively, instinctively. *This* is the behaviour we need to emulate.

I know how daunting this must seem. Perhaps you are still convinced that you need to limit what you eat to stay in control of your weight. And that's fine. Keep doing that for as long as you feel you must. But you do know how it's going to turn out, right? Because that's what you've been doing for decades.

For a moment, let's stop and let the alternative sink in.

How would it feel if all food were allowed? Any food at all. In fact, not only are you *permitted* to eat whatever you want, you *must* eat whatever you want in order to manage your weight.

Try that possibility on for size. Mull it over. Giving yourself full permission to eat anything you like can have a profound and powerful influence on your thinking, your behaviour and your enjoyment of food. When it properly sinks in that you are genuinely allowed to eat whatever you want, something will change in you.

Something will shift.

When all those rules about food are thrown out, and all restrictions are removed, you'll be astonished at how neutral and relaxed you feel.

Possibly for the first time since childhood, you might be able to hear the whispers of intuition. And you may be amazed by what that voice has to say. You'll be astonished at what it wants to eat. All the panic and turmoil about what or whether to eat will be gone. In their place will be a clear channel to an unadulterated sense of wanting or not wanting to eat. A simple, obvious question:

Do I want to eat this or not?

When you give yourself full permission to eat what you want, you'll come to see how often you have been choosing food for some other reason. But now, you'll order the meal you want, without stopping to review the calories, fat or carbs it contains. You'll cook a meal and make it as delicious as possible. You'll add sauces, butter, cheese, breadcrumbs or whatever makes each mouthful perfect, without even a nod towards making it waistline friendly. If you want mayo on your sandwich, you must have it. If you want blue cheese in your salad, have it. If you want a dessert, have it. Eat whatever you want and make it as delicious as possible. If that delicious food happens to be low fat, that is fine. But don't choose the low-fat, low-calorie or diet option because you think it's better for weight loss.

Make no mistake, if you choose 'diet food' because of some arbitrary weight-loss rule, you aren't 'being good', you are actually sabotaging the plan. By not eating what you want, you are ignoring and disrespecting your inner magical wisdom. Only by following this magic action step can you learn to trust yourself to make sensible food decisions *without* outside help.

In time, eating whatever you want will trigger other positive changes in your overall eating habits. The knowledge that you can eat whatever you like will make you less likely to fill up on higher calorie high-carb foods because they don't actually taste of much. You may go off the foods you once thought you loved. Now that you're allowed the pizza, the pasta, the bread and the pastries, you may find they don't have quite the same appeal. But it's only by eating what you want that you'll come to these sorts of realisations.

A CAVEAT: I know that it's not always possible to eat solely what is delicious. We're not always in a position to eat what we fancy at that moment. Sometimes you'll be hungry, and all that's on offer is bland and uninteresting or has been made for you. You might start eating a meal and discover it is overcooked or is too salty. Or maybe your financial situation stops you buying what you really want. So use your common sense here. Do your best. A good rule of thumb is to choose whatever you most want, given the options available.

If possible, and you can afford it, it would be helpful to commit to eating only what is delicious for at least sixty days. This might take more work, more money and more planning than usual. But this short-term financial commitment could pay off massively in the long run. If you can't afford this sort of indulgence, do what you can. Most important is that in this learning period, you get to choose as much as possible, given the foods available to you.

MAGIC ACTION STEP: EAT AS MUCH AS YOU WANT

Having chosen what you really want to eat, the next step is to give yourself permission to eat as much of it as you want.

- *Okay, you've lost the plot now. How can this work? I can eat like a horse. Tell me to eat as much as I want, and I'll literally burst.*

Wait a minute.

I am not saying you can eat unlimited quantities of your favourite food and not gain weight. If you eat twenty chocolate bars and a six-pack of Monster Munch every day, you will probably get fat.

I didn't say 'eat until you explode'. I didn't say 'eat until you feel sick'. I didn't even say 'eat as much as you *can*'.

I said, 'eat as much as you *want*'.

I think you'll agree, when you stuff yourself to bursting, you're not eating as much as you want. You're eating far more.

You're actually eating as much as you *don't* want! If you've ever thought *I don't know why I ate so much when I didn't even want it*, you know what I'm talking about.

Assuming you are someone who regularly or always eats way more than is comfortable, how can the instruction to 'eat as much as you want' help you? How will you know when to stop?

- *Easy! Eat when you're hungry and stop when you're full.*

Yeah, right!

'Eat when you're hungry, stop when you're full' has got to be one of the most useless instructions in the entire world. If it were that easy to control our eating, none of us would have a weight problem.

To help with the difficulty of *eating when hungry, stopping when full*, some weight-loss coaches recommend working with a hunger scale. Using a hunger scale involves rating your level of hunger on a scale of 1 to 10 at various points during the eating process. For example, you would start eating when your hunger level was at 7 or above. You then continue to check your hunger level as you eat. You eat until your hunger level drops to 2 or 3. Once your hunger rating hits 2, you stop eating.

Sounds reasonable, doesn't it?

If you've been successful using hunger scales, please carry on. Sadly, I found working with hunger scales anything but intuitive. Overall, I think they caused even more confusion and second-guessing because I would constantly check and recheck my hunger rating.

Am I hungry enough to eat? Am I at 6, 7 or 8? It's so hard to tell. Should I wait another ten minutes and see if the number changes? Perhaps I'm about a 4 now, or is it lower than that? What IS a 4? I'd better be careful not to eat much more. Oh no, I think I ate to a 1. Did I ruin it all?

Pretty soon, I started using the hunger scale on this supposedly intuitive program as merely another way to restrict what I ate. I'd end up being ultra cautious, putting a tiny amount of food on my plate and stopping eating way before I was remotely full up. The meals got smaller and smaller, and I got hungrier and hungrier because I was so terrified of eating past the right hunger rating. The entire eating experience became about this *number*. All-over body and soul satisfaction didn't come into the picture. And as for accessing my inner wisdom? Forget it! I simply developed a brand new way to feel guilty about food.

Eventually, I'd decide life was too short for all this hunger, counting and numbers. I'd break the diet and, hunger scale be damned, I'd eat for England, Scotland, Wales and the rest of the world, too.

Hunger ratings might be more effective if eating were all about hunger—the fullness or emptiness of your stomach. As we've seen, eating, and in particular overeating, is about a whole gamut of body and soul experiences and emotions that go way beyond mere hunger. If we focus on hunger as the deciding factor in whether we should eat, we ignore a huge part of the eating experience. And given that a lot of the time we're not eating because of hunger, it's not surprising we don't find a hunger scale relevant or helpful.

On this plan, we aren't interested only in physical hunger. We will instead consider a more complete drive to eat—something I call 'pure wanting'.

What do I mean by pure wanting?

Well, babies and little kids, wild animals and naturally thin people find it easy to know when to stop eating because the line to their intuition is clear. They don't have diets, food rules, food shame, second-guessing and confusion about how much to eat interfering with their decision-making. They either want to eat, or they don't.

Their wanting is *pure*.

However, for us serial dieters, there is no such clarity. We don't always know when we're truly hungry, and we don't know when we're full. We often eat way more than we need even when food is not objectively what we want. Our wanting is cluttered and becomes confused as we try to use thinking and reason to decide whether to eat. We have no intuition about food (or at least it seems that way to us).

So, what *is* intuition? As I see it, intuition is an intense trust, a true knowing. We could even say intuition is all you appear to know when you *don't* think.

Intuition about food is the instinctive ability to decide what and whether to eat with no thinking required. What I'm saying is that intuition about food is a kind of *pure wanting*. The simple desire to eat or to *not* eat.

Discovering our intuition about food is undoubtedly the greatest key to overcoming overeating. This will have a critical impact on this entire process of achieving food freedom.

Intuition *knows*. You want to eat, or you don't. There is no second-guessing involved. Intuition helps us to make a decision that is obvious, uncluttered, relaxed and utterly right. It has no need for justification, scientific evidence or rational argument.

Accessing intuition offers such a deep degree of trust that we feel confident in giving up our reliance on diets and third-party experts altogether. We will be perfectly able to eat food of the right types and in the right quantities that will make us fully satisfied, physically and emotionally. Overeating won't even come into the picture.

Ironically enough, restricting the amount we eat is a surefire way of blocking the intuition that tells us we've had enough. By granting ourselves the right to eat as much as we want, we may find we lose some of that compulsion to overeat.

So you see, the only chance we have of connecting with that intuitive sense of pure wanting is by removing all restrictions. We must permit ourselves to eat *what* we want, but also *as much* as we want.

This magic action step can have a radical effect on any tendency to binge. You may even begin to feel, on a fundamental level, that your binges are over. When bingeing, people often eat as fast as they can or eat without thinking because they don't want to listen to the voices telling them *this food is not allowed, don't eat too much!*

But now, there is a clear, sensible voice telling you *everything* is allowed, and *as much as you like*. So you no longer need to gobble down food as quickly as possible so that you get it eaten before your better judgement kicks in. The mindless stuffing isn't necessary anymore. From now on, all food is allowed, always and forever for the rest of your life. And the knowledge that you can have it later takes the urgency out of having it all now. After all, when you have the rest of your life to eat ice cream, why would you feel compelled to eat it all *now*?

We're almost at the end of the first strand. Let's remind ourselves of those first two magic action steps. This entire first strand has been focussed on showing you the vital importance of these two instructions.

1. EAT WHATEVER YOU WANT
2. EAT AS MUCH AS YOU WANT

Incredibly, because these steps begin the process of opening the channel to your intuition, by following them, some of you will begin losing weight, even without the rest of the plan.

But these steps alone won't work for all of you. In fact, some of you would actually *gain* weight if you followed only the advice in this strand. So don't stop here. To have the best chance of success, you must use these first two magic action steps in conjunction with the rest of the book.

STRAND TWO

BEHAVIOURAL TRICKS

Chapter Fifteen

Practical Tips to Prevent Overeating

This second strand is all about the easy, practical steps that can be incorporated into your day. These will effectively prevent the overeating that may occur were you to follow the advice in the previous strand all by itself.

In some ways, this strand may appear to be the least magical of the program. Don't be fooled by its simplicity. The practical steps I'm about to explain will have a profound effect on your eating habits and give you a whole new appreciation of food.

As we have seen, one of the main reasons we overeat is that we aren't getting satisfaction from our food. This is why we must eat exactly what we want.

But there's another reason we may not get full all-over satisfaction from our food, and that is simply that we eat too fast and don't pay enough attention to the experience. For some of us, lack of attention may even be the main reason we overeat. It is also the easiest thing to overcome.

Have you noticed the extent to which we are encouraged to speed up every aspect of food preparation and eating? The faster, the better, in fact. We rush shopping for food, getting it over with as soon as possible, using the fast checkouts, and even ordering online from our phones. We rush cooking food, with quick recipes, 'fifteen-minute meal ideas' or even paying for a delivery service that provides precut and measured ingredients. We also have instant noodles, instant porridge, instant soup, instant gravy, instant coffee and instant custard. You can even get tea that brews extra fast (because let's face it, waiting for tea to brew wastes so much of our day!).

We also rush eating. We may eat on our way to work, or at our desks, working right through our lunch breaks with a fork in one hand and a computer mouse in the other. We grab a sandwich while rushing between meetings, or we gobble down a snack while the children are napping. Because of this, we end up seeing food and the entire act of eating, not as a priority, but as a secondary undertaking to be fitted in around other more important activities.

Even when the food in front of us is hot and home cooked, lovingly prepared, and waiting to be savoured, we may still stuff it down rapidly, with little chewing. From the first bite it can be like a mad dash to the end of the meal, eating so fast you barely notice the experience of food. The meal may be delicious, but you eat so fast you don't much notice it going down. And before you even realise it, you've eaten far too much.

If you're someone who eats like this, you might find yourself at the end of what was supposed to be a delicious meal still somehow empty. You're full, but you're not *satisfied*. You may even start looking around for something else to eat.

The same thing happens when you eat mindlessly. Mindless eating happens when your attention is elsewhere—playing with your phone, working, Facebooking or reading magazines.

It's common to reserve your most delicious meals for sitting in front of a good film on the television. It may feel you are doubling your pleasure by doing two enjoyable things at once. But with so little focus on the actual eating, the experience doesn't have much of a chance to register moment by moment, and there's no chance of getting full, all-over satisfaction. The result is you eat more.

In short, the simple truth is the faster and more mindlessly you eat, the *more* you will eat.

MAGIC ACTION STEP: PAY FULL ATTENTION TO THE EXPERIENCE OF EATING

So, let's move on to the first magic action step of this strand.

There is an easy, almost effortless way to reduce the amount you eat. This is to eat slowly and carefully, squeezing every scrap of enjoyment out of every meal.

Of course, not every meal can be a gourmet extravaganza, but almost every eating experience can be improved by taking time to enjoy it. Even eating a sandwich at your desk will be more enjoyable if you pay attention. The more time you spend eating and the more attention you give to the experience, the more satisfaction you will get from the act of eating, and you'll find yourself eating less without any conscious effort or restriction.

It works this way because every enjoyable experience is subject to the law of diminishing returns. This refers to the way a pleasurable thing gets less pleasurable the more you do it. If you've ever bought a ridiculously expensive bottle of wine, you'll know the first sip tastes fantastic, like nectar. But after a glass or two, it tastes like plain old wine. The first bite of chocolate, or the first strawberry tastes amazing. The first time visiting a beautiful waterfall or forest can be an almost blissful experience. But the fourth bite of chocolate, the fifth strawberry, the eighth time visiting that same waterfall has begun to feel a bit samey. The delight wears off. The return diminishes. Eventually, there comes a tipping point, after which a pleasurable thing becomes no longer pleasurable at all. After five bars of chocolate, two pounds of strawberries or three bottles of wine, there is no enjoyment whatsoever. In fact, the pleasurable thing has become rather unpleasant.

Now, here's the thing: when you rush your food or pay little attention to the experience of eating, that natural tipping point comes much, much later. You eat right past it without noticing. You may have had enough ten minutes ago. But you're paying so little attention, you miss the signals telling you to stop eating. By the time you realise you've had enough, you're already in 'discomfort' territory.

If instead, you slow down, paying full attention, you'll end up getting more satisfaction and more enjoyment out of the entire experience of eating. The result will be that the natural tipping point comes sooner. You'll recognise it easily and stopping eating when you've had enough is automatic and effortless.

This becomes even more powerful when combined with the first magic action step—*eating what you like*. Thus, by

1. eating only what is delicious and

2. paying full attention to eating it,

you could massively reduce the amount you eat with no conscious restriction at all.

What follows are some practical suggestions for making it easier to pay more attention to the experience of eating. Try to include at least a few of these actions every time you eat. Some may be difficult in a public place, but they should all be easy to do at home.

Sit down at a table to eat.

Wherever possible, commit to eating sitting at a table, with cutlery laid out and napkins on the table. I realise a dining table, napkins and even cutlery won't always be available, which is why I say 'wherever possible'.

To get the full experience of satisfaction, you need to be wholly present to the entire experience of eating. This means that during a meal, you should be eating or talking to your friends or family. Nothing else. If you read, watch TV or work while eating, this will serve to distract you, and you won't even notice when you've had enough.

I can't deny it's fun to eat in front of a good film, so I'm not suggesting you can never again eat while watching television. But try to keep it as a treat rather than making it the default.

Sitting at a table is going to require effort for those of you who eat in front of the television every night. But make the effort now, and you'll be surprised at how quickly it starts to feel comfortable. If you're someone who always sits in front of the TV while eating dinner, this one move alone could result in your eating significantly less.

Serve up at the table.

If you serve up in the kitchen and carry full plates to the dining table, you'll likely give yourself a bit too much, if only to ensure you don't have to go back for seconds. And if you've put too much on your plate, you'll feel compelled to finish it. After all, we all know how hard it is to leave food.

Instead of serving up in the kitchen, serve yourself at the dining table. Put each different food item into serving dishes, bowls or plates, and place them in the middle of the table. When you start your meal, your plate should be empty.

Serve yourself food in small portions, around two to three forkfuls or mouthfuls at a time. Don't put big piles of anything on the plate even if you are sure you will eat it all. Keep serving yourself small portions of food, taking no more until the first lot has been eaten. There's never a need to take a big portion because there's plenty right in front of you, and you can always serve yourself more.

If you commit to this way of serving meals, you may be astonished at how much less food you end up eating. It will be hard to believe how much you once served yourself.

Make each forkful perfect and delicious.

Don't eat the boring bits first and leave the best for last or you'll feel compelled to finish everything on your plate whether or not you want it. Make each forkful perfect, with the ideal combination of foods or condiments you like best. Make sure everything you put in your mouth is as delicious as you can make it.

Once the food is in your mouth, put your knife and fork down.

The simple act of putting down your cutlery will force your attention to the food in your mouth, giving you the opportunity to fully savour the experience. To make this even more effective, close your eyes while you chew and swallow. By doing this, you will become aware of the taste and texture of what you are eating in a deeper, more nuanced way.

In doing this, you increase the enjoyment you get out of each meal and become satisfied with far, far less food.

You'll find yourself ready to stop eating after a moderate portion, pleasantly full and satisfied, with no need for willpower, self-control or any sense of deprivation.

There is something crucial I need to say at this point. Paying more attention to your eating should result in your eating less food. But it's essential you don't *try* to eat less.

The point is to eat less *without* trying.

On this plan, restriction is sabotage. So don't focus on eating less. Focus on eating.

Don't reduce food. Increase enjoyment.

Eating less will just be a delightful side effect.

MAGIC ACTION STEP: ALLOW YOURSELF TO WASTE FOOD

There's one more magic action step in this strand.

You must allow yourself to waste food.

I know how hard this will be for some of you. As children, many of us weren't allowed to leave the table until we cleared our plates. Did your parents ever say 'if you don't finish your dinner, you'll be eating it for breakfast'?

I was brought up in a household where money was tight, and for forty years, I found it painful to leave even a small amount of food on my plate. Wasting food seemed sinful and throwing away food that could have been eaten was akin to a crime. Restaurants even used to offer prizes like lollies to children who finished their meals because *good children always clear their plates.*

Perhaps most compelling is the guilt we feel at wasting nutritious and expensive food when there are people in this world literally starving to death.

This all adds up to such a strong compulsion to finish our meals that we eat way past enjoyment, ending up uncomfortably stuffed. After all, isn't it better to eat everything on the plate rather than wasting it by throwing it away?

For me, the big change in thinking came when I started to view the notion of 'waste' differently. I came to realise that whether we eat it or throw it away, the food we buy, prepare and serve ends up as waste. When you eat everything on your plate rather than throwing unwanted food away, that unwanted food ends up in the toilet rather than in the rubbish bin, and then in the sewer rather than landfill. Still waste.

For food to fully serve its purpose, it should be savoured, enjoyed. It should nourish the body and warm the soul. So when you eat everything on the plate even when you're no longer hungry so that food doesn't end up thrown away, you have effectively wasted it. ather than having the food serve a useful purpose, you've almost disrespected it. You've forced down food you neither need nor want. *You might as well have chucked it in the bin.* The only difference is that because you've eaten the excess, you end up putting on weight.

This means:

- Food that is eaten just so you have cleared your plate is wasted.
- Food you eat past your natural stopping level is wasted.
- Food you eat because your mother told you never to waste food is wasted.
- Food you eat because there are people starving halfway around the world is wasted.

And to be clear, no starving person on the other side of the world has ever been helped or comforted by you stuffing yourself.

If you don't want to waste food, make sure it fulfils its role as an enjoyable and nutritious eating experience. If not, it's wasted whether you eat it or not.

If you're concerned about general levels of food waste in society, it might help to recognise that always clearing your plate actually leads to *more* wasted food. Think about it, if you're constantly clearing your plate, even after you're full to bursting, you're wasting this excess food in the toilet rather than the bin. Now, whether the food on our plate is eaten or thrown away, it has still been produced, transported, bought, stored, prepared and served. And you'll never stop buying, preparing, cooking, serving and eating this excess food, unless you allow yourself to waste some of it. Let's say you always take and eat six or seven potatoes and you always finish your plate, even if you're already stuffed, because you don't like to waste food. This means you never get to learn that three potatoes might well have been enough.

If next time you leave some of those potatoes on the side of your plate, you get the experience of wasting food. You experience seeing you've taken too much. You get to learn what your natural appetite is. You get to log that experience and learn something—*more than three potatoes is too much*. As a result, you take fewer potatoes next time, so you cook less and eventually, you buy less. By letting yourself leave food on your plate you will learn how much you truly need, how much to cook, how much to serve and how much to buy. Thus by wasting a bit of food now you can avoid wasting mountains of food in the future.

If you like, you can also try a little trick I learned from behavioural scientist Paul McKenna—get into the habit of always leaving something on your plate. It might be a bit of potato or a few peas. But leave *something* so you get used to the idea.

And if you are still concerned about wasting food, I urge you to start composting. These days, I have become so efficient in shopping and cooking that I rarely waste a thing. If food is left over, I compost it. This takes a lot of the remorse out of leaving food.

If you don't have a garden, composting might be more challenging, but many cities have designated places where you can take your organic waste. Some councils will even collect it from your door alongside your rubbish.

So that was Strand 2. I hope you enjoyed those easy, practical steps that will result in your eating less with no forced restriction at all. Just to remind you, the magic action steps for this strand are:

1. PAY FULL ATTENTION TO THE EXPERIENCE OF EATING
2. ALLOW YOURSELF TO WASTE FOOD

STRAND THREE

CHANGING UNWANTED BELIEFS

Chapter Sixteen

Beliefs Create Your World

A well-dressed woman was looking at my shopping trolley with what I imagined was a mixture of amusement and disgust. Was I being paranoid? Surely, she didn't care that I had bought nothing but ice cream, pizza and Danish pastries. Then I saw it, her perfectly timed glance away and towards her own basket full of organic greens and oat milk. There was no mistaking the wave of smugness that washed over her face.

You may have noticed that I've concentrated a lot so far on combating overeating. But not everyone overeats. Perhaps you have a different issue with weight. If you rarely or never overeat, yet still don't have the body you want, this is going to be the section for you.

A hero's journey isn't all seriousness and fighting. There will be lighter moments too. It's time for one of those lighter moments.

Strand 3 is probably the most enjoyable strand of all. For some of you, this will be the easiest too. This fun and extremely effective way of making massive changes is probably my favourite aspect of the strategy. And the things you will learn here will set you in good stead for the main battle to come.

Having a body that looks and feels great is not merely about food. Another crucial aspect of this whole subject is how we speak and think about our food and our bodies. Even if we resolutely follow every guideline, we will find transformation painfully slow or even impossible if our speaking and thinking aren't consistent with what we are trying to achieve.

I want to start this section by exploring an enormous barrier to success. This is a behaviour so habitual we do it without noticing how detrimental it is. I'm talking about the way we judge food, ourselves and the whole business of weight.

The first way we do this is by imposing values on the food itself. I'm not talking about moral or ethical concerns such as animal welfare or environmental impact. These questions are important but are a separate issue. I mean referring to certain food as 'bad', 'good', or 'wicked'. I've even heard sugar called 'evil', and I remember as a tiny child seeing TV ads for cream cakes with the tagline *Naughty but Nice!*

That's just the beginning. It's not exclusively food that we judge as good and bad. It's also ourselves, the people we are.

- *I was terribly bad today, I had vanilla syrup in my coffee.*

- *I've been exceptionally good today. I've only eaten about eight hundred calories.*

- *I mustn't be naughty and have a dessert when we go to dinner tonight.*

- *I'd love some more mayo on my sandwich, but I'm trying to be good.*

I know the embarrassment of standing at the checkout with a shopping trolley full of snacks; it's the feeling of being a *bad person*. I also know the sense of virtue when I have done a juice fast or stood on the scales at

WeightWatchers and been told I'd dropped two pounds; it's the feeling of being a *good person*.

Perhaps worst of all of this negativity is the way we judge our bodies. We may hate our bodies or feel disgusted by them. We look at ourselves in the mirror and say *look at the state of me; why did I have to be so bad?* We see a particular number on the bathroom scales and fall into despair. *Why can't I control myself? I'm so weak. What's wrong with me?*

This is all incredibly destructive. We have categorised food, our bodies and ourselves as 'good' or 'bad' for so long we haven't stopped to question what we are doing. These moral judgements about food and weight produce similar repercussions as do horrendous beliefs such as *I'm not lovable* or *I don't deserve to be happy*. Our happiness and self-worth become tied to an arbitrary number on the scales, to a bit of flab on our stomach or to our less-than-perfectly-smooth thighs.

This is madness. How can one's moral worth be determined by the eating of some sticks of fried potato? Why should we fall into despair and shame because we see a number on the scales or eat two slices of birthday cake? Never mind that we might be great parents, hard workers and loyal friends. All these great qualities are ignored under the 'bad person' label.

There is also a distinctive self-righteousness tied up with food and weight. Weight problems are often blamed on a lack of education about food, with overweight people patronised by the suggestion they are too stupid or uneducated to eat properly. As if they are imperfect, faulty people who need to be follow rules given by clever, educated people. This is not only arrogant and condescending, it's ridiculous. I mean, why would any person, educated or not, need instructions on how to eat? It's like being told we need directions for how to breathe, how to walk, how to love, how to live.

And it *doesn't work*. Far from helping, all this judgement actually hinders our attempts to manage our weight. We've spent our whole lives subject to conflicting rules and moralistic judgement over food, diet, weight and our bodies from people who are supposed to be experts. This has led to self-doubt and even self-hatred about an experience that should be natural, effortless and hugely enjoyable.

These negative messages have been shouting so loudly and for so long it's become impossible to hear the quiet voice of wisdom underneath. No wonder we make food choices that don't seem conducive to our well-being.

We hear these externally imposed labels of 'good', 'bad', 'good for me', 'bad for me', 'diet food', and we accept them. Good means go, bad means stop. This leads us to stop learning. We don't discover for ourselves whether a food actually *is* good or bad for us, because we stopped short at the label with all its moral judgement.

Now, we may well defy the label (by eating the full-fat mayo, the white bread or the second slice of cake), but we do so with self-recrimination and regret. There's no learning to be had. No intuition heard. No wisdom. Just a sense that we did a bad thing.

The problem is not stupidity, lack of education, greed or some moral failing. It's rather that externally imposed rules and moral judgements make a nasty concoction of shame and confusion that obscures our intuition and interferes with our ability to make sound food decisions.

I'm convinced that moralising about food is not simply unpleasant. It's harmful. Whether a food makes us feel good or bad, makes our stomach hurt or not, even whether we enjoy it, all take second place to the notion of it being an objectively 'good' or 'bad' food. This means vitally important *personal* nutritional information—information far more accurate and valuable than anything found in an outside source or provided by an external expert—*is lost*.

No *wonder* we don't trust ourselves. No wonder we can no longer hear our inner wisdom. No wonder we feel we have no intuition about food. We have spent a lifetime drowning out the signals with negative judgements of our food, overruling and silencing the wisest, most perfect authority there is.

THE EFFECT ON ENJOYMENT

When you consume what you have deemed a 'bad' food, you almost certainly do so with a mixture of confusion, apprehension, ambivalence, even shame or self-contempt.

What stories run through your head?

This burger is full of carbs and fat. This ice cream is bound to make me put on weight. I'm spoiling all my hard work. Eating my favourite food is such a mistake; it shows what a weak and uncontrolled person I am!

Now think about the impact this has on your level of enjoyment. How can you fully enjoy your food when all this negative judgement is going on?

You might be eating something truly delicious, but if you've labelled it as 'bad' or 'forbidden', feelings of failure or shame will take centre stage—masking, blinding or distracting you from the full experience of eating.

This means whenever your eating is marred by shame, worry, stress, guilt, second-guessing or self-flagellation, it detracts from the amount of satisfaction you get from your meal, and yes, you've guessed it:

You feel compelled to eat more.

So you see, far from helping us to manage our weight, negatively judging ourselves and our food typically leads to more overeating, less control and more weight gain.

MAGIC ACTION STEP: CHANGE YOUR STORY

We are going to change all of this. This magic action step has the power to make truly massive changes while also acting as a support for all you're doing.

You are going to begin a whole new way of thinking about yourself, talking about yourself and your food and of relating to the world. In place of all that moralistic nonsense and negative judgement, we are going to offer you a whole set of new, empowering and positive beliefs.

Have you noticed that we usually think in terms of words and that there is a constant commentary running through our minds at all times?

Crucially, beliefs appear in the form of words. Think about such beliefs as 'sugar is bad for you', 'women find it harder to lose weight after menopause', 'I have no control around food', 'I'm always overweight no matter what I eat', 'I'm a greedy person'.

It's easy to see how powerful beliefs like these are. And the truth is, beliefs play a far greater role than merely colouring our experience. In *Becoming Magic*, and pretty much all my books since, I teach that the world we see and experience is nothing but a projection of the beliefs we hold at that time. Put plainly and simply—if you believe you are a fat person, being fat is what you'll experience. If you believe you have a low metabolism, having a low metabolism is what you will experience. If you believe it's hard for you to lose weight, *you will find it hard to lose weight*.

On the other hand, if you believe you are a thin person, that it's easy for you to lose weight, that you have a fast metabolism or believe 'I can eat anything and not put on weight', then *you will experience exactly that*. Our words and beliefs are so powerful, I have often described their effect in terms of magic. Hence the title of my book, *Magic Words and How to Use Them*.

If 'magic' sounds too unlikely or irrational for your sensibilities, no problem. We can also look to science for proof of the power of words on the physical world.

You've most likely heard of the placebo effect—the positive impact of a medically inactive substance or treatment. If you weren't aware, the *nocebo* effect is the opposite of that. It's the negative effect of a diagnosis, inactive substance or treatment.

For example, when healthy patients are told they have a medical condition and are treated for it, they sometimes get sick and start displaying real symptoms. This happens even though the 'medication' given to them was plain old chalk, and they had no actual illness in the first place. The words caused them to believe they were sick. That belief was so strong, they actually got sick.

Now, if the placebo and nocebo effects are this powerful, having real-world, physiological consequences in our bodies, it *must* also be the case that your thoughts and beliefs are affecting your body weight. This must be categorically true, given the power of the placebo effect.

Let's look at some beliefs that may be affecting your body. Do any of these sound like you?

I don't overeat, but I'm still always overweight.
I've always been overweight, and I probably always will be.
My mum and dad are both heavy, so I've clearly got a genetic disposition to be heavy.
I can never shift that last ten pounds.
I'm just naturally greedy.
All women put on weight after menopause.
When I go out to eat, I have to have three courses.
I can't resist a free buffet even if I've already eaten. I guess I don't have an off switch.
Once I start eating crisps, I can't stop until I finish them.

There are also more general beliefs related to nutrition and food itself. I'm talking about such beliefs as:

A meal without carbs is missing something.
A meal without meat is missing something.
Meat/grains/beans or dairy are bad for you.
Meat/grains/beans or dairy are good for you.
Fasting is unhealthy for women.
You shouldn't waste food when there are people starving.
I could never offend a restaurant by leaving food on my plate.

What about the stories we tell while eating or preparing food?

This ice cream is fattening.
I shouldn't be eating this.
This broccoli is awfully good for me.
This salt is raising my blood pressure.
I should put more vegetables on this plate.
I'd love more chips, but I'll have more salad because it's better for me.

Can you recognise these are all just stories? There is no measure by which we can judge any of these statements to be true. All the same, there are doubtless some that you believe unconditionally.

The problem with these stories, even the most 'obviously' true ones, is how powerfully they affect our lives, creating and shaping *what* we experience and *how* we experience it. You may believe you're greedy because you eat too much. But have you ever entertained the possibility you're eating too much *because* of that belief? You may believe you're overweight because all women put on weight after menopause. But perhaps you put that weight once you got to menopause because you *believed* you would.

Given how powerful words, beliefs and the placebo effect are, we are presented with another startling implication: if an inert sugar pill can cure disease because we believe in it, then it must be true that beliefs also affect the nutritional properties of food.

In short, if you believe something is bad for you, it will have a bad effect on your body. When you eat food that you regard as healthy, your body will react in a healthy way. And the more strongly you believe something about your food, the more likely that belief will have a physiological effect. Again, this *must* be true, given the power of placebo.

I'm astonished there has not been medical research into placebo and diet. We know people respond differently to particular foods, which prevents a one-size-fits-all model of nutrition. My suspicion is that whether a diet, a foodstuff, an exercise regime or an eating plan suits us is at least partly determined by belief.

Could it be there is no good or bad food, and our beliefs are what make it so?

But hang on! There must be some foods that are good for us and some that are bad. What about sugar? Processed food? How about *poison*?

Okay, I'm not suggesting we can eat poison and be fine as long as we believe it's healthy. After all, every year in the US alone around seven thousand people poison themselves with wild mushrooms they were sure were harmless. And all accidental overdoses happen because drug users are positive the dose they are taking is safe. But given how powerful placebo and belief are in other areas of health and life, it would be inconceivable that what we believe about a particular food doesn't have *some* influence on its physiological effects. I mean, if believing a drug is effective makes it so, why would this not also be true of food?

Are you starting to realise how much influence your beliefs are having on your own weight issues?

So, what's the answer? If we could change the beliefs we hold about our bodies and about the food we eat, our bodies would transform before our eyes. Even if you don't overeat, you could make massive changes by changing beliefs. If you truly believed *I find it easy to lose weight*, that's exactly what you'd experience.

One of the most powerful, effective and quick methods of developing helpful beliefs, creating change and getting what you want is *telling a new story*. Telling a new story is the subject of two of my most popular books, *Magic Words and How to Use Them* and *How to Do Magic That Works*. The technique was instrumental in how I overcame chronic insomnia, featuring in my insomnia-busting book, *The Effortless Sleep Method* and my online sleep course, *Sleep for Life*. It also played a huge part in how I went from poverty to wealth.

To get a grasp of how telling a new story works, I ask you to recognise that the story you tell about yourself, the world, and your experience comes true. It probably feels that you're merely telling a story *about* an external world. But pay close attention and you'll notice you're not merely reporting, you're *creating* your experience with the story you tell. You experience exactly and only the story you are telling at this moment, believing it to be true without question.

We can't help but tell a story in almost every moment with both our spoken words and with our internal narrative. Now, if we are always telling a story, why not choose to tell the story we would *like* to be true?

To do this effectively, you must change the way you speak to yourself and to others. At first, the new story will sound like fantasy or even lies. But with enough time and consistency, your thinking will align with the new story. In other words, you'll start to *believe* the story. And when your belief changes, your world changes in concert.

Let's look at how this might work with some specific examples.

Suppose you firmly believe that

My mum and dad were both heavy, so being overweight must run in my family. This makes it so much harder for me.

How could we tell this story differently? We need to choose to tell a different story that reflects the belief you would rather hold. Perhaps *my mum and dad were both heavy, and I saw what it did to their lives. That's what makes me extra determined to be different.* Try that thought on for size. Could you at least speak as if it were true? It doesn't matter that you don't believe it yet. Speak as if it were.

Here's another belief. *It's much harder to lose weight when you're older. This is especially true for women because all of us will put on weight in menopause.*

Let's retell this story. Perhaps, *not all older people are overweight, and not all women put on weight in menopause. I've decided I'm going to be one of the slimmer ones.*

Again, try the story on for size. It doesn't matter that you don't yet believe it. For now, speaking *as if* this were true is enough.

Let's try another. *When I go out to eat, I have to have three courses.*

We could retell this as *when I go out to eat, I always leave some food on the plate so I get to enjoy all three courses.*

Again, try it on for size. It doesn't matter that you don't believe it. For now, speaking *as if* this were true is enough.

Here's one more belief. *Once I start eating, I can't stop.*

Thing is, you *can* stop. I designed this program to help you find the ability to stop. So your new story could be *this program is connecting me to my intuition around food, so that I always stop eating at the right time.*

Remember, you don't have to have faith in it right now. Belief will come later. For now, just say it. Whenever you're talking out loud or speaking silently to yourself, speak as if that story were true.

It's even possible to retell your life story so that all the difficulties you've had and all the events you've experienced are now part of a perfect path to where you want to be. For example, *I've been overweight my whole life, and thank God for it. Because it's led me here, to discovering my inner intuition, not only about food, but about life. So, I'm eternally grateful for the troubles I've had.*

These are examples. Don't copy what I've written above because that will be pointless. There is a bit of an art to telling a new story. (Which is why I've ended up writing two entire books on the subject.) In short, three things must be true in order to tell a new story effectively. The words of your story must be:

1. chosen by you alone;

2. told *in the moment*, describing how things are *now*; and

3. they must tell a story or support a story you want to be true.

It's up to you to recast your own stories. Coming up with a new story by yourself in your own words will be infinitely more powerful than anything I could tell you to say.

Probably the most common mistake I see is people treating the story as if it were an affirmation or mantra. For example, they may constantly repeat the following words: *I joyfully allow myself to lose weight with ease while eating healthy, nutritious and delicious food.* Can you hear how artificial this sounds? No one speaks like this.

We should be speaking instead *as if* the desired state of affairs is already true. So stories should sound more like this: *I am sure this program is going to work for me. If I stop and pay attention, I KNOW I'll eat less.*

Can you see the difference? You're not simply repeating the phrases and words, you're commenting on life as you see it now, describing things as they actually are, but *as if the new story were true.*

That's why it helps to keep your story along the lines of something that's close to the truth. Don't tell outright lies, because no part of you will believe them. Instead, tell a story that seems like it *could* be true.

For example, don't say *I weigh nine stone* if you know full well you weigh sixteen. Instead, choose a positive way of describing things that sounds like it could be true. It could be, *I weigh sixteen stone, but I feel lighter. I bet I've put on muscle and lost fat.*

Don't say *My mum and dad were both slim* if they both died of weight-related illness. Instead say something like *My mum and dad were both heavy, but bless them, they didn't have the resources I have. I have it so much easier than them. Mum, Dad, I'm going to do what you never could!*

But remember, you must find your *own* words. Keep speaking according to this new story constantly, commenting on the world as if it were true. And this should be done whether talking to others or privately to yourself.

Don't say what you see. Say what you *would like* to see.

Speak, not like the person you're trying to change, but like the person you want to *be*. Act like the person you want to *become*. Don't wait to become a new person. Be that person *now*.

Please don't underestimate the power of telling a new story. Take it seriously. You'll be astonished at the results. To find out more about this incredibly powerful technique for change, do consider reading *Magic Words and How to Use Them*. It will tell you all you need to know to make this work. You can also complete the Magic Words 5 – Day Challenge. This is a fabulous free course I created to accompany or replace reading the book. Just visit this link to find out more https://becomingmagic.com/magicwordscourse

MAGIC ACTION STEP: STOP COMPLAINING ABOUT YOUR WEIGHT AND BODY

This magic action step is to stop complaining about your body and your weight. That means no moaning about your weight, your food or anything related to it. Complaining is actually another form of telling a story—a negative story. And if we create our experience with the story we tell, this must also apply to when we complain. In this way, by complaining, you're literally creating something to complain about.

So don't complain. *Not at all.*

Do not complain about your body. Do not gripe that nothing fits you anymore. Do not grumble because you overate *again*. No more saying 'I look fat today.' No more 'I ate too much, why do I do this to myself?' No more beating yourself up. Don't say you have no self-control. Don't talk about how difficult this all is for you.

When you realise the power you wield with your story, it no longer makes sense to speak in anything but a positive way about your eating, your diet and your body. You'll soon come to see that every unflattering remark you make about yourself, your body, other people or the way you eat is literally creating a complaint-worthy situation. Complaining is still *creating*. But it's creating stuff you don't like. If you continue to complain, change will be torturously slow and difficult. But by changing your words and stories to be more in keeping with the life you want, you'll see rapid change.

If you have any trouble or resistance to this essential step, again, consider reading *Magic Words and How to Use Them* or complete the 5 - Day Magic Words Challenge. (The link to the course is at the back of the book). I also recommend *A Complaint Free World* by Will Bowen.

Chapter Seventeen

Loving Your Body

What do you think of your body? Do you wish it were different? Do you ever feel your body is your enemy? Do you feel disgust or dismay when you catch sight of yourself naked? Do you even hate it?

You may have been doing your best to tell a new story about your food and your eating, but you can't seem to do the same when it comes to your actual body. *That* still seems like something to bellyache about.

Let's be clear.

Feeling shame, disgust or hatred for your own body does not help you lose weight.

Feeling shame, disgust or hatred for your own body *stops you losing weight*.

Complaining about your body is a form of abuse. Self-abuse. Your poor body. Your poor, devoted, hardworking body is like a faithful servant that works night and day to look after you even though you regard it as disgusting, wrong or ugly. And you abuse it and hurl insults at it, taking it for granted, just because it doesn't look the way you want.

You wouldn't dream of treating a servant or indeed, *any* other human being in this way. You wouldn't ever be so cruel and thoughtless as to say these things to another living soul.

So why do you say them to yourself?

If only you realised: every time you do this, you're continuing to experience a body you don't like. If you like to speak in terms of manifestation, you could say you are instructing the universe to give you a body you don't like. This is what you do every time you say 'God, look at the state of me', 'what a mess', 'I look terrible in that dress', 'I feel like a fat whale'. Every time you speak badly about your body, whine about it, or wish it were different, it's going to *appear* to be a body you wish were different. Whether you want to call it placebo or manifestation, it doesn't much matter—when you feel loathing towards your body, you're going to continue to experience a body you loathe.

So why not love your body, and let the universe give you a body you *adore!*

There's a really fun and easy way to change the way you think and speak about your body. Simply feel gratitude for it. Gratitude is such a powerful force for positive change that in the past I've recommended keeping a daily gratitude journal. This practice can be enormously transformative. But there's an even more powerful way to use gratitude that works well for physical appearance. It's a great little exercise you can do every day. It only takes a minute.

MAGIC ACTION STEP: FEEL GRATITUDE FOR YOUR BODY WITH THE MIRROR EXERCISE

To do this, you'll need a full-length mirror, or at least one in which you can see most of your body. To start the technique, stand naked in front of your mirror and look at your body.

Simply look.

Your mind will do its usual business of categorising and judging, criticising and telling stories, focussing on the bits you don't like. I want you to ignore your mind's wittering, as if it were an annoying fly. Just look.

Next, try to feel grateful for your body. Thank it for all that it does for you. Do your best to feel blessed to have this amazing piece of flesh that works efficiently and tirelessly to keep you safe and alive.

To help with this exercise, try imagining the way someone else would see you. Someone who loves you. Perhaps your mother or one of your children or even a pet.

Does a mother look at her child and see its faults? Does she care her child may carry a few extra pounds or have imperfect skin? Of course not. A loving mother will look at her baby and see nothing but perfection.

Even though you may not always treat it with respect, your body has probably served you pretty well so far. So if you can't feel grateful for the way your body looks, at least try to feel grateful for how well it *works*, for how it looks after you.

I started doing this technique of standing naked in front of the mirror last year. After a few weeks, something rather strange happened. I got up from bed and stood naked in front of the full-length mirrors in our bedroom. And rather than flying to an immediate judgement of whether I looked fatter or skinnier (which had been the norm), I simply *saw my body*. It was so odd. It was as if I were seeing my body for the first time. It was a subtle and strange thing, but I was recognising what a functional, well-designed organism it was. I saw the thing that carries me around through life. I saw the skin, the frame, the muscles, and ...

... I liked what I saw.

I honestly liked it. I had respect for this incredible miracle I saw before me. I looked at all the bits I'd been mentally abusing for decades. The wobbly bits, the stretch-marked thighs left over from early puberty. The scar on my leg from slipping in the kitchen as a toddler. The circular white one on my shoulder from the tooth of a dog that bit me. The thick knees and the almost ghostly, too-white skin.

My body was a bit chunky still, but that day it also looked strong and athletic, a bit like a hockey player's body or a swimmer's body. I felt capable and steady and grounded in that body. It wasn't the exact size I wanted, but that had seemed to disappear into the background. It was the darndest thing. And I suddenly felt nothing but immense privilege and gratitude that this incredible miracle I saw before me was all *mine*. I had been given a whole body. What a *gift*!

This technique will feel weird at first, especially if you have spent a lifetime hating the way your body looks. Loving and being grateful for your body can take a bit of practise before it feels true. But over time, it will become much easier.

And you know, if you *can* find a way to cherish the body you're in, there's a reward in it for you, the greatest reward—something amazing, something miraculous. It's a weird magical paradox that I've seen over and over again. To get what you want, you've got to accept what you have. This means, by loving and accepting the body you have now, *you will get the body you want*.

So tell yourself *The way to get the body I want is to be loving and accepting of this one*. This is not a useless flowery platitude—it's a powerful act of magic. If you can be totally, one hundred percent okay with the body you have, you will get the body you want.

If you are still finding this difficult, try something else. Imagine what you would say if I offered you your dream come true in return for one true positive statement about your body.

Do it now. Imagine the perfect body is yours if you can find one true good thing to say about the body you already have. That's how it starts. Find one true positive thing.

Now find another one.

And you're away.

So that was Strand 3. I hope you're coming to see how a simple matter of speaking differently can have an enormously positive impact on this whole body and weight situation. Just to remind you, here are the magic action steps for this strand.

1. CHANGE YOUR STORY
2. STOP COMPLAINING
3. FEEL GRATITUDE FOR YOUR BODY WITH THE MIRROR EXERCISE

STRAND FOUR

FINDING INTUITION

Chapter Eighteen

You Never Really Lost It

Okay, we're on to Strand 4. This is possibly the most difficult part. It is also the most powerful. Everything you've read until now is about to become far more effective, as it's time to inject some magic into the proceedings.

Our tale is approaching the halfway point, and we are coming closer to our main battle. In many adventure stories, there is a moment of calm, of rest and respite before the lead-up to the big challenge. This is the base camp before the final ascent, the friendly village at the bottom of the mountain that holds the dragon's cave.

Before we begin our trip to the cave itself, I need to talk about a rather pleasant subject—the nature of happiness.

In Strand 2, I asked you to recognise that eating is not merely about hunger. We eat to get all-over, body and soul satisfaction. In light of this, I even suggested a craving for ice cream, chocolate or other delicious food could indicate a healthy instinct to abandon a restrictive diet. After the deprivation of a diet, your body doesn't need ice cream, but it's possible your being needs it. Your soul needs it. Your emotional self needs it.

But this isn't the full story, is it? What if this goes too far? I mean, yes, we are not machines needing only fuel. Yes, it's clear that eating isn't always about hunger. Yes, eating is enjoyable and sometimes highly social, and celebrating with food is something every culture on earth has done since the beginning of human history. Yes, we often go off-diet because of a healthy need for body and soul satisfaction. But I can't pretend a grand celebration or reacting to a restrictive diet are the only reasons I've ever overeaten. If I'm honest, they make up a tiny fraction of the times I've overeaten. I have eaten way past fullness, to the point of regret, even when there hasn't been a diet in sight for months. And far from being sociable, I've usually done this alone in my own home.

So how and when does our natural enjoyment of food turn into something else? Why does 'feeding the soul' become 'gorging the body'?

Some use eating as a powerful soothing mechanism for painful emotions. Loneliness, boredom, depression, grief, and hormone-induced moods can be hard to bear, and the compulsion to block out those emotions with food can feel overpowering. But it's not just those with difficult emotional struggles who find themselves out of control around food. The tendency to mask, fix or distract ourselves from uncomfortable feelings is present in almost all of us. Even if that feeling is simple boredom, we may turn to food to banish it. In other words, we eat for entertainment, to distract ourselves, to liven up a dull evening or for no good reason at all.

No matter how much we tell ourselves we shouldn't, we still reach for that fifth, sixth, seventh biscuit. We take enormous portions and go back for seconds. We have a pudding after dinner even though we're already stuffed. And do we *ever* eat chocolate because we are hungry?

Do you often say *I don't even want this. I don't know why I'm eating it.*

So why are you eating it? Think back to the last time you seriously overate. I mean a time when you properly stuffed yourself. Did you eat that way because you were hungry or even because you really wanted what you were eating? Or was it more a case of having some inexplicable compulsion to eat until you couldn't manage another bite?

What induces you to do this?

Why would an otherwise intelligent, sensible person eat until they were sick or in pain?

The answer is you eat this way because you want *something*. You try to sate yourself with food, but because food isn't really what you want, it doesn't work. So you carry on eating, searching for that elusive *something* until you can't eat another bite.

Let's look at this in more detail.

Chapter Nineteen

The Wanting Mechanism

As babies and toddlers, we live totally in the moment. As we become older, developing a sense of self and other, we start to feel separate and scared and begin looking for things to repair this sense that something is wrong. From then on, moment-by-moment experience takes the form of a constant search. We're all familiar with this. I'm talking about the near-constant need for more or different. This might be anything from a deep sense of lack or longing to a vague notion that 'I want *something.*'

It's the sense that this moment, *this one now*, isn't quite right. It could be better. And one way to *make* it better may be to feed it with food. This is what fuels comfort eating. (I'll use the familiar umbrella term 'comfort eating' to refer to all forms of emotional eating.)

If you are prone to comfort eating, it's going to be especially difficult for you to stick to a diet. 'Handy' tips like 'drink a glass of water half an hour before a meal' or 'remember to fill up on vegetables' won't help much since, in truth, hunger isn't the reason you're eating.

Overeating past the point of comfort is nothing to do with hunger. It is an attempt to feel better. It is an attempt to find happiness.

Your endeavours to lose weight through sheer willpower or restriction are almost guaranteed to fail because the *future* happiness that might come from being thinner is eclipsed by the *current* happiness you can get *right now* from eating some delicious food.

We all have the tendency to search for happiness in external sources even if we're not prone to overeating. When this search is focussed around a harmful substance like cocaine or a potentially destructive activity like gambling, we call it addiction.

I've never been addicted to drugs or smoking or gambling. But working? Self-help? Distraction? The need to be doing something? Even helping others became a kind of addiction for me. So let's recognise that overeating is not about greed. It's about comfort. It's about a search for happiness.

In fact, greed doesn't exist. We don't call the workaholic greedy when he works a nineteen-hour day. We don't call the fitness fanatic greedy when she spends four hours in the gym every day. Nobody called me greedy when I was obsessively giving all my money away to charity. Why not? I was just trying to find happiness in something that is deemed socially acceptable, but it's the exact same mechanism in action.

That so-called 'greed' for food is in fact the universal craving for happiness. You have it. I have it. We all have it. Whether it's giving all your money away to charity, eating too much or shooting up heroin, it's the *same mechanism at play*.

So don't beat yourself up over your addiction to food or booze or smoking or drugs, and don't judge others for theirs. Because what fuels their addiction to cigarettes or wine fuels my need to work too much and my obsession with helping others. It's what fuels the need to reach for your phone when you're bored and start scrolling. It's what fuels the desire for bigger and shinier things. It's what fuels the desire for self-improvement and spiritual growth. And it's what fuels much of our overeating.

In fact, it's what fuels almost everything we do.

But there is a problem. *It doesn't work.* We never find true happiness in food (or drugs or booze or overworking). If we did, addicts would be the happiest people on the planet. And they clearly are not. We don't find the happiness we seek, because there is a massive misunderstanding at the heart of overeating, addiction and almost everything we do in our pursuit of happiness.

And now we come to the third key factor in overeating.

OVEREATING FACTOR 3: WE MISUNDERSTAND WHERE HAPPINESS COMES FROM

Have you ever stopped to consider what happiness is or where it comes from? For a start, happiness is not something we can feel in the past or future. We cannot feel yesterday's or tomorrow's happiness. It can only be experienced *now*. We may be happy at the thought of a future event or a past memory, but we *feel* that happiness right at this moment.

Also, you can feel only your *own* happiness. You may be happy when your children or parents or friends are happy, but you cannot feel what they feel. You can only feel *your* happiness here and now.

How strange then, that we spend most of our lives focussed, not here and now, but *there* and *when*.

'I will be happy *when* ... '

It's the unwitting motto of almost everyone on the planet. We live in this body, this here, this now. But we spend almost our entire lives focussed somewhere else—on the past and future, on places and times that happiness *cannot be felt*.

And here's where it gets mysterious. If I'm experiencing happiness at the thought of a future event, what causes that? When I feel good having just received a gift or when I'm in good company or in a beautiful place, where does that contentment come from?

It's natural to think that the source of happiness is that gift, that company or that beautiful place. We are happy, it seems, because that gift, that circumstance, those people *make* us happy. Thus we assume that happiness *comes from* ideal circumstances, being with our favourite people, and getting what we want.

Or it comes from the right food. When we get that first bite of delicious food, there is a rush of bliss. It feels amazing to get that first square of chocolate or that first spoon of ice cream or that first glass of cold white wine on a summer's afternoon. We feel happiness! And it seems as if the food or drink has caused it.

But it's an illusion. That's not how it works at all. Happiness is not something that comes from getting what we want, even though it *really* looks that way. It is not something that comes from any part of the outside world. It's not something that comes from past or future. And it's not something that comes from food. All that happens when we get that first bite of mouthwatering food is that the background yearning, that search, the subtle wanting that's there almost every second of our lives *stops* ... for a few moments.

The pleasure that comes when you get something you want is the *absence of wanting*. Happiness is the exquisite state of not wanting for anything. That's what happiness is. It is nothing inherent in the food, the drug, the drink, the lottery win or in any part of the outside world.

Happiness is identical with the absence of wanting.

They are the same thing.

Now, the sense of well-being that comes when the wanting drops away doesn't last, because the search fires up again almost immediately. And because you assume that it was food that caused the good feeling, you reach for more. Even when you stop enjoying the food, your 'wanting mechanism' pushes you to eat more because that's where it thinks the happiness comes from.

Whether it's saying you won't be happy until you eat a pizza, get a boozy drink, pay off all your debts, find a husband or get ten thousand likes on your Instagram post, it's the same mechanism. Even if the message is you'll be happy when you can help others or when you get over your depression or when you can eradicate world hunger—it's the same mechanism. And it is never satisfied because none of those things is a source of happiness. That's not where happiness comes from.

The irony is that every time you get something you want and feel happy, it feeds into the illusion that 'happiness comes from getting what you want'. You think you're making yourself happy by getting things, creating things, achieving things, when all you're doing is feeding that addiction to wanting, searching for more or different. This is why the search never ends.

There's a rather strange consequence to all of this. You may have a good idea of what you want: lose weight, find a partner, get rich, buy a house, overcome a problem, get some spiritual growth or whatever. But *that's not honestly what you want.*

Wanting is a search for happiness. Happiness is a ceasing of that search. So what you are truly seeking is an end to the seeking.

You want an end to the wanting.

So, when we crave food, what we actually want is for that craving to stop. Whether you crave pizza or vodka or an end to inequality, in reality what you long for is for that craving to stop. Because that's the one time you feel happy.

You can feel happy and free only when there is no wanting because that's what happiness *is*.

You see, indulging in food doesn't give you happiness. It doesn't give you anything; it takes something away. It takes away *wanting*, if only for a little while.

So why does this matter?

Because it means if we want to be happy, we don't need to go anywhere, achieve anything or search for anything. We surely don't need to *eat* anything because happiness is already here now. Not in the world, not in the drugs, not in the booze, not in the food but in you. You don't have to go anywhere to get it. It's here now.

I know this might be difficult to swallow, so let's try to prove it. Get some of your favourite food and allow yourself to crave it. Feel the strength of that wanting. Recognise the discomfort in that yearning. Then, take a bite of that food and feel the experience of happiness. Pay close attention and see if you can sense where that happiness is coming from. You'll notice that the wanting falls away as you eat. It evaporates, leaving something behind.

Left behind is happiness.

It isn't created or produced—it is *revealed*. Your innate, eternal happiness reveals itself when the wanting that was covering it up disappears.

And here's the best bit. There's another, better way to access your innate happiness—one that doesn't involve food or booze or anything external.

Once you realise this, you'll discover it never was food causing happiness in the first place. And when you know that overeating is not bringing you any joy, you'll have no compulsion to do it. No willpower will be required.

It won't make sense to look for happiness in food because you'll know, deep down, that no happiness will be found there.

Overeating will never look attractive again.

THE THREE KEY FACTORS IN OVEREATING

Everything we have heard so far about overeating can be distilled down to these three key factors.

1. No contact with intuition

2. Lack of satisfaction

3. A misunderstanding of where happiness comes from

If we can attend to these three things, we will have no need to worry about what or how much we eat. Notice I have said nothing about a need for willpower or self-control. This is perhaps the most delicious and magical part. We learn to stop overeating *without* needing willpower. We really do get to dump the diets, *permanently*.

Unsurprisingly,

1. contacting our intuition;

2. getting full satisfaction; and

3. understanding where happiness really lies

are inextricably linked.

If we can contact our intuition about food, we'll know *what* and *how much* to eat. We'll eat just the right food to make us perfectly satisfied, both emotionally and physically. And because we're getting so much satisfaction from the food we *do* eat, we no longer feel compelled to eat so much of it.

In the process of contacting our intuition, we'll also discover the true source of happiness. As a result, we'll no longer have any need to use food for comfort alone.

The result will be a calm, easygoing freedom around food combined with so much satisfaction from the act of eating that there will never again be a need for restriction of any kind.

This is the entire premise of this plan.

Chapter Twenty

But What About Physical Addiction?

Before we go on, I feel I need to address this topic for the benefit of anyone concerned about the physical, biological processes at play in many addictions. Drugs like heroin, nicotine and alcohol and even things like sugar and chocolate have a chemical makeup that makes them physically addictive. This suggests there's a lot more going on with addiction than a misunderstanding, lack of satisfaction or lost intuition.

It's true, there is a physically addictive quality to foods like coffee, sugar and other carbohydrates. This is largely down to the withdrawal effect that compels us to want more. This is a chemical, physical, biological thing. It's real.

Having said that, it's astonishing how the enormous power of the mental addiction exceeds the tiny effect of this physical addiction. With drugs like alcohol and even heroin, the emotional aspect definitively outweighs the physical addiction.

Consider the twelve-step program with its premise, 'once an addict, always an addict'. Even decades after consuming the last bit of alcohol or drugs, an addict may still need meetings, commitment, willpower and constant effort to prevent the relapse that is almost inevitable without this ongoing support.

And this is *years* after all traces of the drug are gone from the system. Those weekly meetings are necessary to fight the *mental* addiction, not the physical or chemical addiction. If addiction were exclusively a physical or chemical problem, no one would ever relapse once the drug or nicotine or alcohol was out of the blood. No recovering heroin addict would ever go back to the drugs, no alcoholic would still need to go to AA ten years after the last drink, and no sugar addict would reach for chocolate again months after last eating it. Sadly, plenty of addicts *do* relapse, even after many years.

A family friend, Eddie, was a serious alcoholic in his twenties and thirties. Aged thirty-six, he gave up the drink with the help of AA and a lot of therapy. That was forty years ago, and he hasn't touched a drop since. Good for him.

Recently, my mother asked Eddie if he ever craved a drink. His response was, 'I crave the drink every second of every minute of every hour of every day!'

Poor chap. Eddie is still addicted, despite forty years without a drop of alcohol in his body. He beat the physical addiction half a lifetime ago, but the mental addiction is still there decades later because Eddie still believes that booze has the power to make him happy.

Given this, we can see why addiction is such a problem.

No matter what steps we take to abolish the addiction, such as twelve-step programs, diets, willpower or abstinence, as long as we believe that a bit more happiness lies in the drink, or in the fix, or in the food, we will continue to crave it. And if we don't attend to the causes of our craving for the substance in the first place, we cannot beat the addiction. Little wonder that AA asserts 'once an addict always an addict'. If you haven't taken steps to come to terms with the feelings that led you to drink in the first place, you still *are* an addict.

What I'm saying is different. I'm saying that because we all have that same wanting mechanism, in a sense, we are all addicts.

But we don't need to remain that way.

If we can find a different way to deal with the feelings we are trying to escape by eating, we will no longer try to cure them with food. And if we can access the *true* source of happiness, we will stop looking for it in food, drink, drugs or in any part of the outside world.

BEGINNING THE INVESTIGATION INTO FEELINGS

We have seen that a misunderstanding lies at the heart of the tendency to eat to feel better—we think we are finding happiness in food, when actually the good feeling comes from within us.

On its own, this information doesn't help us. We can tell ourselves *this craving for chocolate is a misunderstanding*, but we still eat too much of it. Thus, we may know, rationally, that this food will not make us happy, nonetheless, we find ourselves stuffing our faces with it *again and again*.

This shouldn't surprise us. Overeating involves acting *contrary* to our rational judgement, eating more than we need—more even, than we *want*. Reasoning with ourselves is never going to help because an intellectual, mental, rational understanding isn't what we are looking for.

Overeating is not a rational thing. It is an emotional thing. It is a *feeling* thing. We overeat to *feel* better. So forget rational argument. Forget trying to convince ourselves of the truth. We need a deeper, gut-level understanding that happiness isn't found in *more* food. To get the experiential, visceral understanding we need, we must go straight to the heart of the issue—*to our direct experience of feelings themselves.*

This is where we will find that elusive pure wanting. This is where we find the ability to make clear, uncluttered decisions about what to eat, and whether to eat at all. The raw, direct *feeling* of this moment is the doorway to your intuition.

And through this doorway is where we're going next.

***

We are approaching the key point of our hero's journey. We are ascending the path that leads up the mountain to the dragon's cave. There's no turning back now.

The challenge is near.

Chapter Twenty-One

The End of Suffering, The Discovery of Happiness, and The Rebirth of Intuition

Let me ask you something. *What do you feel right now?*

Maybe you're in a good frame of mind because you've had a great day or heard some excellent news. Perhaps you're stressed or worried about money, or a family member or the economy. You could be pissed off about this, that or the other. Or perhaps you feel that life is going well.

In short, if you report what you feel, you will undoubtedly start telling me a story. You'll give me reasons and an explanation for the way you feel.

But that's not what I asked.

I didn't ask *why* you feel the way you feel. I asked *what* you feel. Notice the way your natural inclination is to move immediately from the feeling itself to the explanation, to all the circumstances, the real-world issues affecting you, and the apparent *reasons* for the way you feel. If you experience a lot of troubling emotions like anxiety, sadness, loneliness or anger, you probably spend more time focussed on thoughts *about* the anxiety and *reasons for* the anger than actually feeling them.

We all do this with apparently good reason. When we aren't eating our troubles away, we are thinking or talking about why we feel bad. We do this because it distracts us from the direct experience of the bad feeling itself. After all, it's easier to talk about anxiety and sadness than it is to live through them.

Thinking, talking and eating aren't the only methods we use to avoid emotional pain. Almost all forms of therapy, treatments and methods for dealing with painful feelings are different ways of correcting how we feel.

Anxiety medication works to dull or sedate fear. Antidepressants work to counter unhappiness, 'filling in' the apparent serotonin gaps. Even relaxation techniques often contain the implicit assumption that *I must soothe the bad feelings away. What I am feeling is wrong. I must find a different, better, more relaxed feeling.*

And, of course, many of us eat. Eating is a tremendously easy way of fixing feelings because it's something we all do every day anyway. It's never hard to find an excuse to eat. Eating never eliminates our pain for long, but in the absence of anything better, we turn to food again and again.

Whether we choose eating, medication, therapy, drinking, watching excessive TV, doomscrolling or playing video games, the underlying motive is the same. We are trying to avoid feelings we can't bear to feel.

And it's totally understandable. We avoid disturbing feelings because we don't want to suffer. But ironically, and tragically, this is precisely why we suffer so much.

Here's why: Sadness, anger, fear, boredom and even physical pain are not suffering. Even grief and deep shame are not suffering. Suffering is our *resistance* to these feelings. Suffering is the extent to which we judge them as wrong.

You know that sense of needing to push them away, run from them or fix them? *That* is suffering. That *resistance* is what feels so deeply uncomfortable.

Resistance *is* suffering. And suffering *is* resistance.

They are identical.

Of course, to soothe this suffering, many of us choose to eat. We eat, we comfort eat, and we *over*eat, all in an attempt to fix the way we feel.

It is frustrating that when we fight the urge to eat, this sets up another level of resistance, another level of suffering. The more we fight or control that craving to eat, the worse we feel. And the worse we feel, the more we seek relief in food. This is what happens in a spiralling binge when the shame of the binge itself leads you to eat even more.

Every attempt to fight the urge to binge, and every story telling you how you must resist the craving, and every scrap of self-recrimination about how bad or shameful you are leads inevitably to more and more discomfort and more likelihood you will overeat to escape it. It's a vicious circle. A trap.

There's but one way out.

We need to stop running. Stop trying to escape. We need to go *in*. We need to go *through*. Not away from the feeling, but *towards* it.

It's time to *feel* those damned feelings here and now.

The truth is feelings don't need to be escaped or fixed. None of them. Not even the worst anxiety or sadness. If we can find the courage to stop avoiding uncomfortable feelings and instead to fully experience them, an amazing transformation will take place.

By feeling deep into this moment, *particularly* when you are suffering, you'll discover that most of the suffering was coming from your *resistance* to those feelings, not from the feelings themselves. All suffering is resistance to what is here now.

And astonishingly, when we stop resisting and feel through our discomfort, we don't suffer more, *we stop suffering altogether.*

***

We have now reached a critical stage of our hero's journey.

You are now effectively standing at the entrance to the cave. In the cave lives a fearful monster, an enemy. But it's an enemy you must face if you are to come home with the treasure of transformation. The enemy is fear, shame, disgust, anger and every disturbing emotion we can feel.

It's time to go where you don't want to go, to feel what you've been too afraid to feel. It's time to stop running and face up to the job. It's time to be a hero. If you want to find the treasure you seek, you must enter the cave you fear to enter.

Ready? Then let's step inside.

Chapter Twenty-Two

Introducing The Hero's Process

We are so used to trying to avoid or fix certain emotions that it has never crossed our minds to do anything else. Even if we wanted to, most of us don't know *how* to feel what is here right now.

I've devised a simple process to help you do precisely this.

I call it the Hero's Process.

The Hero's Process is a method by which we learn to feel what is here now, making no effort to change or repair it. Thus:

We don't run from fear. We *feel* it. We don't distract ourselves from boredom. We *feel boredom*. We don't cheer ourselves up when we feel sad. We *let ourselves feel sad*.

It may seem paradoxical or even outright wrong. But please don't dismiss this or assume it doesn't apply to you. Allowing yourself to feel discomfort without trying to change it is possibly the most transformative thing you will ever learn.

Mastery of the Hero's Process will give you confidence and control over your eating, but that's just the start. The process will help also with your mental health and resilience, your ability to deal with stress and your general levels of happiness and contentment. It helps eliminate anxiety, depression and to overcome insomnia.

It may look like merely another version of 'fixing feelings', but that's not the case at all. The Hero's Process is more like a fundamental way of relating to your experience. It's almost a way of being. Once understood and mastered, this process will change your life.

Now, there are many ways you can use the process. But I have identified three slightly different versions for the purposes of this book.

1. Use the *Hero's Process* whenever you feel anxious, angry, upset, sad, worried or have any strong, unpleasant emotion.

2. Use the *Hero's Process* to help decide whether and when to eat.

3. Use the *Mini Process* once or twice during a meal to help decide when to stop eating.

I'm going to start by taking you through the full Hero's Process for dealing with strong, upsetting emotions like anxiety, depression or shame. This will be a longer, more detailed explanation to show you how the process works.

Next, I'll explain how to use the Hero's Process to discover intuition about whether and what to eat.

And finally, I'll show you how the Mini Process can be used midmeal to prevent you eating more than you want.

In truth, all these versions are the same process, differing only in the depth of application.

It will take a little while to go through the process the first time. I'll be giving a lot of explanation and guidance as I go so you can see in detail how it works. But once you're proficient in using it, you'll be able to use the process quickly even while you go about your daily activities.

I have also created a free downloadable MP3 recording of the Hero's Process so that you can listen rather than read. Just visit

> https://www.becomingmagic.com/feasting-resources/

MAGIC ACTION STEP: USE THE HERO'S PROCESS ON ANY STRONG, UNCOMFORTABLE FEELINGS AND EMOTIONS

Now, it would be great if you could try this out when you are experiencing a strong, unsettling emotion so you can play along in real time. If you don't have any troublesome feelings right now, work with whatever is here. So, let's do it. It's time to be a true hero.

Stop and close your eyes if it's safe to do so.

Next, take three deep breaths, exhaling fully. As you breathe, tune in to your body and notice the rising and falling of your chest as the breath enters and leaves your body.

Now ask yourself what you feel.

There may be an obvious sense of something like boredom, confusion or irritation, shame or sadness. Notice also that stories and thoughts and reasons will pop into your head to explain the way you feel. *I'm irritated because I don't want to do this now* or *I'm stressed because I've got too much work to do* or *I'm worried because my rent is late*. There may also be thoughts and judgements about me and this process. Can you see there is a feeling *and* a story about that feeling? There seems to be a feeling and an explanation for it at the same time.

However, none of these observations are our concern because that's not what we're looking for. The label or name of the feeling doesn't matter. We're not interested in what it's called or even whether you know what the feeling is. No matter what the thoughts are saying, ignore them. Direct your attention away from your thinking, and just drop into your body.

What we're interested in is a physical, bodily sensation.

I want you to ignore everything your mind is telling you, all the stories, labels and reasons, and go straight to the in-the-body sensation of whatever uncomfortable emotion is here. Ignore every thought. We are interested only in the sensation *itself*.

To help with this, try scanning your body for any sense of tightness or a gripping sensation. Is there a fuzziness, a churning? Is there an emptiness, a fluttering, or a discomfort anywhere? If so:

Where in your body is the feeling located?

Direct your attention there.

If you have trouble with this, place your attention in your chest, your stomach or your throat and feel what is there. (Years of sleep therapy consultations have told me this is where the majority of people experience most of the feelings.)

The only thing we're interested in is a physical sensation. When you have found a place where there's a sensation of some kind, whether it's pleasant, unpleasant or kind of neutral, *that's the feeling to work with*.

And if you feel a strong discomfort, maybe anger, shame, sadness or some other unwanted emotion, *don't back off*. You're about to do some magic.

Whatever the sensation is, notice it for a moment. Just let it be there.

Next, I want you to push that sensation away. Try to push it right out of your body. Say a big, internal *No!* to the sensation. Fight it, force it out as best you can.

What happens?

Doesn't it feel worse when you do that? Isn't that interesting? The feeling gets more uncomfortable when we try to get rid of it.

Now, try saying *yes* to the feeling. Nothing else but a big, internal *YES!*

What happens?

What feels different when you do this? It's a little lighter, isn't it? Maybe a little more peaceful?

From there, see if you can gently welcome the feeling. Just as much as you are able. Accept that the feeling is here and acknowledge it. Allow it. Be with it for a while. Let it be okay that it's here.

What happens when you do this? Can you notice an easing, a relaxing, a loosening of the grip? Even if you notice only a tiny lessening of the feeling, that's good. We can now move on.

Next, move slightly towards that feeling and gently allow yourself to feel it.

Now feel it a little more.

Now feel it a little more.

And a little more.

Allow yourself to feel that sensation as much as you are able. And then, if you can, drop right into the heart of the sensation and feel the totality of it.

This is the absolute key moment of our hero's journey. This is how we overcome the monster. We defeat the sensation by allowing ourselves to feel every bit, by letting it flood our bodies until there's no resistance left.

The sensation that started out so uncomfortable has now opened up, lost its tightness, sort of thinned out. You may also feel a bit happier or more relaxed. You might even feel a sense of release, like an ungripping, relief, a lightening or a sudden dropping away of a weight you have been carrying.

That's the shift we're looking for.

Now, if you're frustrated because you don't understand what I'm talking about, you're probably trying too hard. That's fine. It's not a problem. All you need to do is relax into the physical in-the-body sensation of frustration at not knowing what I'm talking about. Feel the physical tension when you try hard to understand. This is not a mystical experience; it's incredibly ordinary. It's not an intellectual thing—it's a bodily experience.

If you feel very strong resistance to doing this, feel into that resistance, feel into that fear. If you are anxious about doing this, feel the anxiety. If you are irritated by what I'm saying, feel the irritation. If you are frustrated that you can't 'get' this, feel the frustration. If you don't have a clue what I'm talking about, *feel* that sense of not having a clue. Always work with whatever feeling is here.

Now, it's possible you will feel some extreme emotion during this process, especially if you've had a lifetime of pushing your feelings down. In my experience, these powerful emotions are usually grief, with floods of tears, or anger in the form of consuming rage. But you might also feel something else: shame, guilt or despair. If the emotion is overwhelming, back off for now and return to it another time. There's no need to force yourself.

But if you can find the courage to face it, do so. Do your best not to run away. This awful feeling has been locked away for years. Hidden, suppressed, but not gone.

By feeling it, you will let it be free. It will express itself in the most perfect way. So don't suppress any urge to cry or rage. If you want to cry, cry. If you want to shout, shout. But keep on feeling what's there.

I promise you this, when you are ready to fully face the dragon of strong, uncomfortable emotions, your life will change. There is magic on the other side of that pain. But the only way to overcome the dragon, the one route out of the suffering, is *through* it. What we fight grows stronger. But what we allow transforms into light.

In time, I this process becomes enjoyable and starts to feel instinctively right. You will be happy to allow the whole intensity of *any* feeling to wash through you, to let it fill your whole body.

There's no set time for how long you should do this. But ideally, you would continue this process until any disturbing emotion has drastically lessened and you are relaxed and happier. But any shift is good. The important thing is to keep allowing and feeling and allowing and feeling at least until something seems to 'shift', and you feel different. This could take as long as five to ten minutes when you first try it. But in time, it will take less than a minute.

If you like, you can repeat this entire process until you feel total peace. That *will* happen if you keep going.

In the beginning, there may only be tiny shifts in the way you feel, but take great delight knowing that every bit of fear, sadness or anger you release in this way is gone for good. In time, you'll feel markedly different. You'll have a thoroughly new experience of life, plunging into the heart of deep, dark fears with a spirit of adventure, just to see what's there.

Chapter Twenty-Three

Using The Hero's Process to Discover Intuition About Food

It might have felt like a diversion to go off into talking about dealing with anxiety, depression and deep shame. I mean, what does this have to do with food freedom and losing weight?

The Hero's Process isn't useful only for handling emotions like shame or anxiety. It's also a doorway to intuition about food.

You see, your direct experience of this moment holds a fundamental truth that only you can access. It feels the way it feels. The raw, direct, immediate experience of this moment does not lie to you. You might think *about* the way you feel in different ways. You might argue about how to describe what you feel or what name to give it, but you cannot doubt *how* it feels. This is the one source of information you can trust fully.

And here's where it gets interesting.

By allowing yourself to feel whatever feeling is here, you will eventually find yourself somewhere rather fabulous. A still, quiet place sitting beneath the discomfort. The present moment. The here and now.

This is where intuition lives.

Here, instead of craving, conflict and confusion, we find a sort of relaxed intelligence. A calm, decision-making ability. We no longer need to follow what others tell us to do, because it is obvious.

We no longer need to engage in an exhausting mental tussle regarding food and whether to eat, because the decision is remarkably straightforward. We discover the utter simplicity and obviousness of pure wanting—the genuine desire to eat ... or the lack of it.

Finally, we rediscover our intuition about food!

This mysterious 'now' is more than a place that feels nice. It's the seat of your intuition. It's the place from where you can make all the right choices about what to eat and in what quantities. The perfect, innate ability to eat right, for you.

Now let's apply this Hero's Process directly to food.

A great way to illustrate how the Hero's Process helps us find intuition about food is to take you through using it for strong food cravings or any powerful desire to eat.

The basic process of facing and feeling through discomfort will be the same as previously explained. But this time, I have placed the Hero's Process within a step-by-step formula specifically applied to food.

Let's start by asking a question.

Do you ever have cravings for certain foods? Do you even perhaps have 'trigger foods', such as chocolate, crisps, cookies or other treats that you feel out of control around? Are there some foods you find so irresistible that once you start eating them you find it awfully difficult to stop?

For example, you could have a real issue with an ice cream craving, perhaps sometimes eating an entire litre tub in one evening. Or you might have a chocolate addiction that leaves you powerless to stop until the bar is finished. If this sounds like you, it may appear you have no option other than to impose a blanket ban. *No ice cream for me, ever. No chocolate for the rest of my life.* This is exactly what some therapists and psychologists recommend.

But there is a problem with banning our favourite food—it doesn't stop us wanting to eat it. We still want it. We are simply denying ourselves the pleasure. We are using willpower to fight the craving. This means we are still under its power. And as long as this is true, there's always a chance we'll cave in to the craving and eat a whole freezer full of ice cream, a six-pack of crisps or an entire family-sized chocolate bar. Or even two.

We have been led to accept that craving is something that must be fought, denied, squashed or avoided with distraction tactics like brushing your teeth or drinking a glass of water. It must be replaced with nicotine patches or gum. In the case of heroin, it must be mitigated with other, slightly less addictive drugs such as methadone.

However, if we regard craving as something that must be fought or avoided, we will never truly be free of it. When you fight a craving, it doesn't go away. It's still there somewhere, waiting to pop back up, possibly even stronger next time. If we do fall off the wagon and indulge in this 'forbidden' food, things only get worse. Having lapsed and failed and broken our promise, we find ourselves in negative self-judgement, guilt, shame and confusion about what to do next. Shame and guilt are strong and unsettling emotions that effectively block our innate wisdom about when to stop and when we've had enough. Thus, in the long run, a blanket ban on our strongest trigger foods may result in the total opposite to the desired result, because one little indulgence of the trigger food is far more likely to turn into a full-blown binge.

Plus, not everyone has a particular food craving. Some people, including me, tend to crave eating in a more general way. I have most definitely referred to myself as a food addict in the past. But I have never had a danger food like chocolate or crisps. I often would crave fish and chips, or a sandwich, or a Sunday roast or a curry or chicken stew and dumplings, or just *food*. A blanket ban can't work for people like me, because we can't ban *food*.

Now, before we start, we need to acknowledge something. It may feel that what you crave right now is a bar of Cadbury Dairy Milk chocolate. But that's not actually what you want. You don't crave chocolate. You don't even crave food. Remember, the happiness we are all searching for is equal to the exquisite feeling of the falling away of wanting. So, what you are truly craving is for the feeling of the craving to *stop*.

So, let's make it stop.

MAGIC ACTION STEP: USE THE HERO'S PROCESS ON A FOOD CRAVING OR STRONG URGE TO EAT

You should use this process every time you feel a powerful craving to eat. And when I use the word 'craving', I'm not referring only to that sort of strong, ravening desperation for chocolate or sugar. I mean any powerful desire for food. What I'm about to show you applies equally whether you have a craving for a particular food or whether you have a more generalised craving to eat *something*. So, if you don't have a specific trigger food but often crave food more generally, this will still be hugely helpful.

Sometimes you may not be sure if you're hungry or thirsty or just bored. But don't concern yourself with these differences. If you have a strong desire to eat, that's all we need to know. That's what we're going to work with.

And one last important point: Don't omit the process because you know you are definitely genuinely hungry. Do it anyway.

So, let's say we have a maddening pull to eat right now. What exactly do we do?

Step 1. Stop.

First, we stop, and we pause. It need only be for a few seconds, but this pause is a thing of power. This is an act of heroism in itself. At this pause, we take control. We acknowledge that we have a choice. This time, we will not let things run on autopilot. In a sense, we are setting an intention: We are doing this thing, and we are committed to doing it properly. We are effectively girding our loins before going into battle with the dragon.

The next stage is surprising.

Step 2. Give yourself permission to eat.

Remember, we use intuition—not arbitrary rules—to make eating choices. Unless there is a known health reason, you always have full permission to eat whatever you want. If your doctor has told you not to eat something, then obviously don't. But otherwise, it's imperative that no foods are banned. You are totally, one hundred percent allowed to eat anything, even if it's your worst, most addictive trigger food. However, giving yourself permission to eat obviously won't work by itself, and I implore you to be a grown-up about this. Don't read 'you have permission to eat whatever you want' as an excuse to stuff your face. You'll obviously end up putting on more weight. To make this work, you must follow all five steps listed here before eating.

Step 3. Do not indulge the craving.

The third stage is crucial. You must *not* indulge the craving. Every time we indulge the wanting mechanism by eating, we feed the mistaken belief that happiness lies in food. We need to show this up for the lie that it is. This means refusing to do what the wanting mechanism is telling us to do.

The magic of this stage is to let that craving be there without feeding it. By doing this repeatedly, the belief that *this food will make me happy* will eventually break down.

- *Hang on right there! I thought this plan was about no restriction or willpower. And now you're telling me to fight the craving, to resist the desire to eat.*

I'm actually suggesting the opposite.

I never said you must fight the craving or the yearning for food. I said don't do *what the craving is telling you to do*. You have full permission to eat this food, but not *while* you are craving it. The time for eating *is* coming. It just arrives a little later.

The real magic emerges when we move on to the fourth stage of this process.

Step 4. Use the Hero's Process.

Let's now address the maddening sensation of the craving itself. If you give in and eat to ease the discomfort, you end up reinforcing the pattern and fuelling the food addiction. So instead of dispelling the craving, either by eating or by fighting the desire to eat, we are going to *feel* it.

Feelings are there to be felt. So, let's jolly well feel them!

You are now facing the dragon. The time to be a hero is upon you. But it is not a battle you are facing, it is not a fight you are entering, it is far scarier than that. It is the total acceptance of that which you dislike.

The choice is yours. Will you distract yourself, run from it, hide behind a rock or avert your gaze? Or will you have the courage to look the dragon full in the face?

The dragon is nothing but a craving.

This craving is nothing but a feeling.

All we need to do is *feel* it.

I'm talking about feeling that craving *as* craving. That wanting *as* wanting. We must take the hero's way through and feel the full force, the height, the strength, the pull, the peak of that craving without doing anything to get rid of it. We must fully experience that sensation, in all its intensity, *without eating*.

We are not battling, resisting or denying the craving. We are not going cold turkey. We are doing nothing but feeling right through the peak of that sensation of craving, without eating. Right through to the other side.

Through allowing yourself to feel a craving, you'll find it will lessen or even disappear altogether.

Once the craving has passed its peak, you can move to step 5.

Step 5. The question

Once you've felt that shift in the way you feel, once any extreme craving has vanished or diminished, there's one more thing to do. You must ask yourself a question, and you must answer it honestly.

What do I really want?

The answer may surprise you. You started this process with a strong desire to eat in order to feel better. But you may be surprised to find you now want something quite different—entertainment, love, happiness, peace, rest, home, connection or company—and the idea of eating no longer appeals.

If we were craving food to escape strong, uncomfortable emotions, we find something incredible happens. Now that we have *felt* the emotion that was causing us to eat in the first place, the desire to eat disappears. Why would you eat when you aren't hungry? Why would you eat when what you want is entertainment, relaxation or to talk to someone? How is food going to give you company? It can't and it won't. You'll be able to see this quite clearly now, and instead of turning to food, you'll feel a natural, obvious compulsion to do something different. You might pick up a book, watch a film, have a bubble bath, call a friend. You may even get a burst of energy and go for a walk or do a fun activity.

Overeating avoided!

You may even discover you want *nothing at all*. You may find yourself doing nothing but sitting in the bliss and peace of not wanting anything.

However, here's the really good bit:

You may find that what you actually want is *food*. Not a maddening craving, but a genuine need for sustenance. A natural, calm desire to eat.

If that's what you find, great!

You've discovered pure wanting. You have connected with the intuition within you. This is the part that never makes a mistake. If it's telling you to eat, you can trust it and move on to step 6.

Step 6. Eat.

At this point, you can—and *should*—eat safe in the knowledge that you have discovered a genuine desire for food. So, eat. Enjoy. Savour.

Can you see the difference here? Eating in this way means you never give in to a craving. You respond only to a genuine desire to eat. Hence no addiction, no pattern—merely a sensible, healthy decision to eat something delicious. The beauty of the Hero's Process is that it means never needing to use strong willpower to battle or overcome food cravings. All we need is the determination and commitment to

1. Stop.

2. Give yourself permission to eat the food.

3. Do not give in to the craving itself.

4. Do the Hero's Process until the craving passes or lessens.

5. Ask yourself what you really want.

6. Eat the food if you still want it.

That's it.

So, it turns out we need a teeny-weeny bit of willpower—just enough to allow the feeling of lack to be present without trying to fill it or fix it with food. But compared to the willpower needed to fight the craving or the self-control needed for a strict diet, this amount of effort is tiny. And we don't need to do this forever. The point is to weaken that craving mechanism enough to enable us to 'see through' it. Just enough to learn that *when I feel like this, more food is not actually what I want.* Just enough to feel this truth at the level of the gut. So, make no mistake, resisting food will become effortless. But we need to make a bit of effort now to get to that place of effortlessness.

As you work with the process, you may discover deeper and deeper levels of sensation and emotion that you didn't even know were there. This may feel like things are getting worse. This is common and is actually a good thing. It means repressed emotion is coming up and out. This is all fine. The full depths of your craving and emotional discomfort may reveal themselves only once earlier levels have been felt and released. If your food habit is long-standing, you should not expect it to disappear immediately. It might take repeated attempts to release it completely. So don't worry for now if some craving or discomfort seems to still be there. And rest assured, when any disquieting feeling or craving is fully felt and released, it's gone for good.

But now that you have full permission to eat whatever you like, how will you make sure you don't eat too much of it? Once you've discovered a pure wanting for food, how will you know when to stop?

I want to introduce you to the Mini Process.

The Mini Process is a short and simple version of the main Hero's Process that takes exactly one minute to complete. You can do it whenever you don't have time to do the full Hero's Process. But it's also a great way of tuning in partway through a meal to determine whether you've had enough to eat.

MAGIC ACTION STEP: USE THE MINI PROCESS TO PREVENT OVEREATING DURING A MEAL

To Do The Mini Process

1. Stop eating. Put your cutlery or food down (this is important).

2. Tune in to the feeling in your stomach and body. Feel whatever is there.

3. Wait one full minute while eating nothing.

4. Ask yourself 'Have I had enough? Am I still hungry? Do I want any more?' These are not difficult questions.

5. The answer is *yes* or *no*. Answer honestly.

6. If you want to continue eating, do so.

7. If you've had enough, stop eating.

8. Repeat two to three times during a meal.

To stop *when you've had enough*, all you need to do is pay proper attention to the way you feel and ask yourself 'Have I had enough?' No need to overthink it. In fact, there should be practically no thinking involved at all. It's thinking that complicates these questions. So, ignore your mind and go with your gut.

If you do this as directed, you'll be sated far, far earlier than you might expect. And you'll find yourself stopping after a moderate portion—happy, pleasantly full and satisfied. Stopping for one full minute and asking 'What do I want?', 'Do I really want this?', 'Do I actually want any more?' is extremely powerful. That pause alone could make all the difference. Even if you don't buy into the whole Hero's Process, you don't feel you have contacted your wisdom and you don't honestly get this whole 'feeling your feelings' thing, simply pausing to follow the Mini Process in the middle of a meal can have a really positive impact your overeating.

However, whether we choose the Hero's Process or the Mini Process, we are *not* using it as a device to reduce the amount we eat. This is extremely important.

We are not using the process to *make us eat less*.

We are using the process to find out *if we want to eat at all*.

Eating less is a side effect. It is not the point. The process is applied to determine whether there is a genuine desire for food. If you focus on eating less, you'll end up restricting your eating, essentially sabotaging what we are trying to do here. It doesn't matter how much you've eaten or how many calories you think you have already consumed, if you find you still want to carry on eating after going through the steps, then *you should carry on eating*.

Chapter Twenty-Four

The Awesomeness of The Hero's Process

The Hero's Process is the foundation on which the entire plan sits. It is the glue that holds everything together and increases the effectiveness of every step. This one practice added to your day has the power to change your entire relationship to food, your body and your weight.

The Hero's Process will always put you directly in touch with your own inner wisdom. No matter what is going on, what your thoughts are telling you or which temptations present themselves, if you feel into the craving or desire to eat, you will find the voice of intuition. It will always be there, and it cannot get things wrong. This technique enables you to know, to *really* know from the depths of your innate magical wisdom, *what*, *when*, and *how much* you truly want to eat.

The Hero's Process is effectively the sword with which you slay the dragon, the magical weapon you wield to destroy all enemies. But unlike a sword, this weapon commits no violence. Nothing dies and no one is hurt. The power of this weapon isn't in deadly, murderous might, but in acceptance, welcoming and gentleness. The Hero's Process is almost a weapon of love. And when the fight is upon us, we go into a loving, accepting, almost *surrendered* battle.

This Hero's Process may sound simple. And it *is* simple. The Hero's Process is merely the action of moving towards uncomfortable feelings rather than trying to fix them.

And being perfectly honest, I don't claim to have invented the idea. Plenty of other authors, gurus and coaches over the last several thousand years have recommended leaning into discomfort rather than moving away from it.

However, I think the fancy name I've chosen is apt. What I'm suggesting is a radical idea that runs contrary to the way the entire world is set up and the way most people run their lives. Moving *in* rather than *away* is counterintuitive, sometimes unnerving and actually rather heroic.

We spend our whole lives trying to change, correct or control the pain, the suffering, the loneliness, the guilt, the hurt, the shame, the craving. All of them painful feelings we try to dispel with external distractions and events, with medication and therapies.

And for most of us reading this book, with food.

But it's all wrong. All of it. Every time.

Nothing in the external world, including food, will ever fix a bad feeling, because that's not how feelings work. The best that can happen is that something in the world will distract you from the pain, but it cannot cure it or alleviate it.

That's why the Friday night binge never actually works to make you feel better, even though it seemed like such a good idea at the time. It merely acts as a temporary distraction, as a deadening of the pain. So the moment it's over, the bad feelings return—this time with an added dose of remorse and shame. We could have avoided this whole situation by doing one thing—the only thing you ever need to do about an uncomfortable feeling: feel it. Without judgement, resistance, complaining or commentary.

If you feel lonely, don't eat your way out of it. *Feel the loneliness.*

If you feel afraid about a future event, don't eat to numb the anxiety. *Feel the fear.*

If you feel shame at a past event, don't block it out with food. *Feel the shame.*

If you feel bored, don't seek distraction in ice cream. *Feel the boredom.*

If you feel something is missing from your life, don't mindlessly munch through crisps in front of the television. *Feel that feeling of something missing.*

If you feel nothing but a mad craving to eat until you pop, then *feel that mad craving.*

If you feel confused or frustrated that you don't know what I mean, *feel that confusion.*

No need to label the emotion as fear, shame, boredom, confusion. No need even to *know* whether it *is* fear, shame, boredom or confusion. Don't analyse or give explanations. This is just more pointless story. Just feel it. Without the story—simply the raw, real bodily sensation of whatever's here.

Without the addition of a story, feelings are just feelings. Some are nicer than others, but without the story none is overwhelming or unbearable. And having felt them fully, you'll know that any desire to eat is coming from a healthy and sensible desire for food in that moment. A neutral, happy, healthy desire.

With time and practice, you'll start to realise on a deep level that you no longer need to battle, fix, or drown out any anguish with food. You'll find that by feeling your feelings, there is no longer any need to eat to escape them. Instead, you can allow them to express and flow through your body back to the nothingness from whence they came.

Food freedom will be yours.

That's the end of Strand 4, the densest and most difficult of all the strands. I admit, that was a lot to get through. You should find the rest of this plan quite easy in comparison. Remember, you can also download a free MP3 of the Hero's Process by visiting https://www.becomingmagic.com/feasting-resources

Before we leave this strand, here are the magic action steps you should take to rediscover your intuition.

1: USE THE HERO'S PROCESS ON STRONG, UNCOMFORTABLE EMOTIONS
2: USE THE HERO'S PROCESS ON A STRONG URGE TO EAT
3: USE THE MINI PROCESS TO PREVENT OVEREATING DURING A MEAL

STRAND FIVE

DISCOVER YOUR OWN PERSONAL
NUTRITION EXPERT

Chapter Twenty-Five

Your Inner Food Guru

So, what about nutrition? I'd like to start by stating I have nothing whatsoever to say about the merits or dangers of any individual food. I don't claim to be an expert in nutrition and I'm certainly not an expert on your body. I don't know what food is best for you. But somewhere, deep down, *you* do.

I'm taking it as a fundamental truth that a human being is capable of making nutritionally correct food choices. If this weren't the case, it would mean that human beings, unlike all other animals, are faulty when it comes to choosing and eating food. This would imply that we are basically broken as a species, having lost the ability to properly feed ourselves.

I don't accept that. And I hope you don't either.

I put it to you that under the messed-up thinking about good and bad foods, under the changing government guidelines and faddy diets, under the food industry propaganda, under the confusion and second-guessing, under the indecision and recrimination, under the body shame and guilt, under the fear and loathing lies the perfect knowledge of *what* to eat, in what *quantities*, that provides all the nutrients for the health of your body *and* your soul. That perfect intuitive knowledge is in there somewhere. We're going to find it and let it speak.

If we are to learn what foods suit our bodies, we may need to let go of many of the rules we have blindly accepted about nutrition. Third-party food rules aren't necessarily wrong. But when it comes to your body, the cleverest nutrition guru on the planet can't hold a candle to the wisdom of your own personal experience.

For example, I know I am moderately intolerant to most bread, but not pasta. I can eat croissants but not rye bread. I don't feel good eating lots of red meat, and bacon always gives me a tummy ache. Raw onions make me fart. Garlic makes me burp. Sugar has no obvious effect of any kind unless I've already eaten a large meal, in which case it makes me terribly bloated. Beans, lentils, rice and root vegetables all feel nice in my belly. I have something approaching an allergy to any kind of beer (it gives me an instant headache) but not wine or spirits. Champagne makes me happy. Vodka makes me heavy and depressed. And more than two glasses of any alcohol makes me feel terrible the next morning.

These things I know. But how do I know? This nutritional information came not from doctors, dieticians, celebrities, TV or medically endorsed whatnots. It came not from government guidelines or information leaflets. This knowledge came from noticing what does and doesn't feel good in my body. No doctor, nutritionist or other adviser could have given me this information. Why would I listen to an expert or follow a rule rather than heed this personal, individual, perfect knowledge of what food suits me?

My mother, my sister, cousins and nephews are all severely lactose intolerant. None of them learned this from a leaflet telling them dairy is bad for you or from a fitness guru promoting vegan diets or even from consulting a doctor. They learned it by noticing how they reacted after drinking milk.

Let me emphasise I'm categorically *not* telling you to ignore your doctor's advice on diet. I mean, if your doctor has told you 'Eat less sugar or you're going to get diabetes', you would do well to listen. If you've had your gallbladder removed or have celiac disease, keep following medical advice! But if your dilemma is whether to eat beans or wholemeal bread, whether to be keto or vegan, you might do better listening to yourself.

You may well decide to eat a plant-based diet. You may decide to avoid sugar. You may decide not to eat processed meat or white bread. But this no one's business but yours. It is a matter for you, your conscience and your body to decide.

- *What if my body tells me to eat cake? How can it ever be right to eat cake?*

I'm not suggesting cake is good. Neither am I saying it's bad. The cake exists. That's all we can say. Take away the moral judgement and all you have is flour, fat, sugar and eggs. Simple, natural foods. Food is food. Any judgement of it as 'bad' sits floating above reality like a malevolent genie. It does nothing but add an unpleasant smell to the situation. I don't care if it's sugar or fat or ice cream or steak or macaroni cheese. It's not good or bad. It's just food. Now when it comes to this irresponsible cake, maybe you *do* react badly to the gluten or the sugar. You might well feel sick if you eat too much. But you'll know when not to have another slice, because of the way your body *feels*. You know that gluten or sugar doesn't suit your body because *you've noticed it for yourself!*

In order for us to make sensible, personal, informed decisions, food needs to be seen as nutritionally neutral until we discover its effects on our individual bodies. Let's start that process of discovery now.

MAGIC ACTION STEP: EXPERIMENT WITH LOTS OF NEW FOODS

We probably all have some idea of what foods do and don't work for us. But what if we don't? What if we don't know where to start, with no idea what foods suit our bodies?

After decades of ignoring our natural wisdom around food, we may have a lot of relearning and discovering to do. So at least for the first sixty days, we will go back to the beginning. To discover from scratch what does and doesn't make us feel good, while also learning more about what we do and don't like. To do this, we'll need to experiment and have fun with lots and lots and *lots* of new and unfamiliar fresh and home-cooked foods.

This step is particularly important if you are used to eating a lot of food that you sense is probably not very good for you. Busy people often eat a lot of processed or takeaway food even though they feel rotten after eating it, because it's quick and requires little effort to prepare. This is not a ban on sugary or processed food. If your intuition is telling you to eat pizza, then pizza is absolutely right for you in that moment. But if all you ever give your body is pizza, you don't give it the option to choose something else.

Trying unfamiliar food seems to go against the rule to eat only what's delicious. After all, chances are you won't like some of those new foods. The thing is, if you confine yourself to your usual meals, you may miss out on foods you and your body will love. If what you count as delicious is only sugary, processed food or if you have a small list of go-to ingredients, you will need to widen your diet to discover new foods that your body might require.

Here we find another, perhaps unexpected reason for overeating—if we eat food that is lacking in the right nutrients, our body may compel us to eat *more* in order to obtain that missing nutrition.

For example, have you ever been to a party buffet, and it's full of 'beige food'—pastries, crisps, sausage rolls, cakes—and you stuff yourself stupid even though none of it tastes very good? And then when you get home afterwards, even though you're over-full, you feel compelled to eat more, to eat something else, something wholesome, something real?

A similar thing may have happened when as a child you ate chocolate for breakfast at Christmas. After a morning of poor nutrition, you needed 'real food' and you were *so* ready for that Christmas dinner!

I'm not suggesting there's anything inherently bad about chocolate, pastries, crisps or sausage rolls, or *any* food. But when you eat processed, premade food or you eat a meal that's lacking in the right nutrients, it's almost as if your body doesn't recognise it as food. And so, because it doesn't find the nutrients it needs, your body pushes you to eat more and more, trying desperately to find that missing nutrition. This is one reason why when you eat processed or fast food, you tend to eat so much of it.

So, you're going to need to try new things in these first sixty days. Experiment with unfamiliar foods or those you wouldn't generally consider eating. Maybe aim to try one new food each day. If you do this, you'll almost certainly discover a taste for things you'd never have considered before, foods you never imagined you'd like. I mean, if you've never tasted black olives and feta cheese in a salad, or fresh parsley with tabbouleh, or toasted sunflower seeds or roasted cauliflower, you're in for a treat. And if you are someone who *detests* vegetables, try chopping them into small pieces before roasting them in the oven with a spray of olive oil, salt, pepper and herbs. Almost every vegetable tastes incredible prepared this way. And the difference between free-range, organic meat and factory-farmed, mass-produced stuff is ... well it's enough to make you want to never go near that cheap stuff again. Yes, it's far less expensive. But when you pay attention to how it tastes, you may find you'd rather eat a small amount of good quality, ethically reared meat than huge amounts of the crap stuff every day.

MAGIC ACTION STEP: USE THE MINI PROCESS TO DISCOVER YOUR PERSONAL NUTRITION EXPERT

When trying any new food, it's important that you take into account the way it makes you feel during the meal and the way it makes you feel afterwards.

To do this, use the Mini Process in the following way.

While eating something new:

1. Put your cutlery or food down (this is important).

2. Tune in to the feeling in your stomach and body. Feel whatever is there.

3. Ask yourself *Am I enjoying this? Is this delicious?*

If the answer is yes, notice that. If the answer is no, notice that.

After eating, do the same.

1. Tune in to the feeling in your stomach and body. Feel whatever is there.

2. Ask yourself *Did that meal make me feel good?*

If the answer is yes, notice that. If the answer is no, notice that.

By doing this, you will be in a much better position to judge what is and isn't right for your body, noticing any digestive issues, any mood changes, any decreased or increased energy. You will discover what you truly love to eat, but you will also discover what your *body* truly loves to eat. If you do this process correctly, at least much of the time, these two aspects—health and desire—will agree. And if they don't—for example, you adore bread but it makes you bloat—it doesn't mean you can't ever eat bread again. But the choice to indulge or not will be *your* decision, made in the moment, based on your knowledge about taste and effects.

If you are used to certain foods being banned because you are liable to overeat them, you may find it impossible to imagine that your taste and your body can agree. If you have ever made yourself sick by wolfing a whole tub of ice cream in one sitting, you are familiar with the experience of eating something you truly love but that your body doesn't.

- *Yes, I hate 'healthy food'. If you let me eat only what's delicious, I'll live on pizza and ice cream.*

I challenge this. If you paid close attention to the way you feel, you'd discover that eating *only* pizza and ice cream makes you quite uncomfortable and not at all satisfied. Maybe you'll always adore ice cream, but by allowing yourself to eat it, paying attention to the experience, and feeling into your body while you eat it, you'll discover you don't need to eat as much to be fully satisfied. When it comes to any delicious food, you'll find that most of the tastiness and genuine enjoyment comes from the first few bites. By savouring those few mouthfuls and letting that deliciousness register, you'll find yourself easily able to stop once that initial yumminess has been and gone. As a result, you'll end up eating *less* ice cream, yet astonishingly, enjoying the experience far *more* than if you gobbled down a whole tub of it without thinking.

Hence, mind and body in full agreement.

As time goes on and your intuition grows, you will feel less and less tempted to eat things that don't suit you. You'll find you aren't as drawn to foods that make you feel bad. You won't need to consult this year's government guidelines, this nutrition authority or that one. From now on, you will have your own perfect, custom-made, firsthand wisdom to call upon. This means when you crave foods that don't suit your body, it's no longer a choice between total denial and a mindless, guilt-ridden binge. From time to time, we all enjoy things that don't make us feel good, be it a glass of wine on a school night or a third slice of birthday cake. And from now on, with the full knowledge that a favourite food doesn't really suit your body, you are free to decide whether to eat it. No rules. No pangs of conscience. No recrimination. Just a deliberate decision based on your own personal evidence.

So, you won't abstain from bread because a YouTuber told you to do it. But you might give up bread because it's not worth the tummy ache you know you'll get afterwards.

BE PREPARED FOR YOUR TASTES TO CHANGE

Following this step can have a surprising consequence. You may come to realise that favourite foods don't do it for you anymore. The foods you once thought delicious don't taste as good. You no longer mindlessly eat a whole family-size bag of crisps because after six or seven crisps they aren't that enjoyable. White carbs may taste so incredibly bland and give you such awful bloat that you stop taking a mountain of potatoes, pasta or rice.

You'll also discover a taste for things you might not expect, and this could happen without you even being aware of it. Vegetables may come alive with flavour, while junk food may come to taste unbearably sweet or salty. You may start eating more healthily with no conscious effort.

Case in point: For most of my life, the biggest, baddest 'banned' food was always KFC. Of all the salt-ridden, ethically challenged junk foods, KFC is the one that has always tempted me the most. Even when I was a strict vegetarian, KFC still called to me. I hadn't given myself permission to eat it in years, but it continued to haunt my dreams ...

... until recently.

On starting this plan, I gave myself full permission to eat anything I wanted, including KFC. Right now, I could call Uber Eats and get KFC delivered in half an hour. But now, praise be to goodness, I don't want it anymore! I mean, why would I eat something so salty, so messy, so greasy? Why would I eat something that makes me feel so rotten, that makes me burp and bloat? Without even tasting it, my KFC obsession appears to be gone!

Similarly, all my life, I've been what you'd call a carbohydrate addict. I've never had much of a sweet tooth, but I have always been a huge fan of bread, pasta, potatoes and mountains of rice. My favourite meals were always pasta, dumplings, roast potatoes and my favourite lunch was the British staple—a sandwich and a packet of crisps. But when I started paying proper attention to the experience of eating these things, something amazing revealed itself. These simple white carbs are dull, bland and uninteresting. It's hard to eat much without feeling heavy and over-full. And that sandwich-and-packet-of-crisps lunch? I might as well eat a whole newspaper or a cardboard box for the way it makes my stomach feel.

I still eat carbs with almost every meal but a small fraction of the previous amounts. A tablespoon or two is usually enough—not because I'm trying to be good, but because that's all I want.

A year ago, I'd have told you I hate salads. I've always enjoyed cooked vegetables, but raw veggies, leafy greens, cucumber and celery? Nasty, hard cold things. I couldn't see the point. But over the course of this plan, I have discovered a previously unheard-of desire for fresh crunchy salads with red onions, beetroot, toasted sunflower seeds, black olives and fresh mint. Salad is somehow no longer cold and hard and raw but tastes fresh and alive and clean. It's not only that these salads taste good. They also feel good in my tummy, leaving me settled and satisfied. I now eat fresh salads almost every night, and my body seems to love me for it.

Interestingly, I have almost without noticing also drastically reduced my alcohol intake. For most of my adult life I was a classic British binge drinker. I didn't drink very often, but *when* I drank, I drank a *lot*. The hangovers were so brutal that in the past I used willpower to refrain from drinking for long periods of time. I'd always end up going back to it, not because I craved the alcohol, but because I somehow felt I was missing out on all the fun.

How strange then, that I have found myself drinking less (in fact, I'm now close to teetotal) without even knowing quite when it happened. I mean, we all know that too much booze causes hangovers. But for most of my life, the link between booze and being happy and celebratory was strong enough to win out. The pull of 'happiness lies in another drink' was irresistible.

But for some time now, I've been paying very close attention to what and how I eat and by association, what and how I *drink*. And the link between 'too much booze' and 'feeling terrible' has been forged so powerfully, the desire for alcohol can't win out anymore. Now I *only* associate booze with feeling awful. So why would I drink it?

For me, giving up the booze has been an unexpected benefit of my paying attention to what I put in my body, and it happened without a scrap of effort.

You can become similarly comfortable and stress free around food *and* drink by paying close attention to the way it makes you feel. Get used to eating what *your* unique and perfect body wants and needs. You can stop eating too much, and you can stop eating things that aren't right for your body. Not because a doctor has told you, not because you feel guilty, but because *why would you do something that doesn't feel nice?*

So that was Strand 5. Let's just remind ourselves of the magic action steps for this strand.

1: EXPERIMENT WITH LOTS OF NEW AND UNFAMILIAR FOODS
2: USE THE MINI PROCESS TO DISCOVER YOUR PERSONAL NUTRITION EXPERT

In Strand 6, we're going to speak about something highly magical, perhaps unexpected but totally necessary.

Let's move on to that now.

STRAND SIX

LETTING IT ALL BE OKAY

Chapter Twenty-Six

How to Deal with Mistakes

So far, we have been working to rebuild trust in yourself and get you in touch with your natural intuition about food. Eventually, you'll trust yourself, confident in your ability to choose the right food in the right amounts. But this ability won't come overnight, and you're unlikely to get it all right straight away. In fact, in the beginning, it might feel like you're getting it all wrong.

In the early days, you might eat more than you want and end up too full. You might eat something that doesn't agree with you and get a tummy ache. You might inadvertently tell an awful story about how fat you look and bemoan your inability to lose weight.

And that's fine.

MAGIC ACTION STEP: GIVE YOURSELF PERMISSION TO MAKE MISTAKES

Try to accept that it's absolutely all right that you make these sorts of mistakes. Let everything be okay. For goodness' sake, don't beat yourself up, declare you've ruined everything or call yourself a greedy idiot. That will set you right back.

We've all fallen into negative stories. Most of us have complained about our bodies. And nearly every person on the planet has occasionally eaten more food than is comfortable. Why add negative judgement, self-recrimination and hair-shirt-donning after the fact? These little slip-ups are opportunities to stop, reflect, learn and move on. But they are never a reason to rebuke yourself.

It's extremely important to be okay with occasionally eating too much. If you fall into despair over an instance of overeating, you'll end up starting another faddy diet on Monday. You'll then be back on the yo-yo, the rollercoaster of dieting, restriction, loss and gain, starving and bingeing, control and loss of it. And the instinctive mind that *knows what to do* is once again silenced, drowned out by the mountain of fuss, rules, confusion and blame.

Without negative judgement, a bit of overeating results mostly in a full tummy and a lot of belching. But it means nothing. Without the negative judgement, there's no pattern, no habit, no *Here I go again, what's wrong with me?* So, let's set aside the self-flagellation for now. *Let everything be okay.* It's all, *always* okay.

I mean, what sort of person do you want to be? Are you going to fall into despair and beat yourself up over a little slip-up? Or are you going to pick yourself up, acknowledge you did something not in keeping with who you want to be, and learn from it?

Consider how a child learns to walk. Can you imagine saying to a toddler who stumbles *You clumsy idiot, you've fallen AGAIN! Why can't you walk in a straight line, for goodness' sake?* You'd never say that to a child.

Or think about learning to play the piano. In the early days, you might press a wrong key. And the clank of a wrong note will sound out. Do you call yourself a stupid, uncontrolled, tone-deaf fool who can't be trusted?

How good a piano player would you become if this were your thinking? How natural, how intuitive, how confident would you feel around that piano?

I want you to view relearning to eat in the same way as learning to walk or learning to play a piano. Eating a bit too much of something or eating something you don't really want is no worse than taking a stumble or pressing a wrong key. It's not a moral failing. Nothing is ruined as long as you get back on track and learn from the experience.

In fact, these sorts of mistakes (so-called) can be enormously valuable.

Learning to play the right keys on a piano *requires* learning how it sounds when you press the wrong ones. And the way to discover what's right for your body will involve sometimes eating things that *aren't* right. And let's face it, the only way to discover how much is enough is to occasionally eat too much.

I regularly make this point in my work as a sleep therapist. I tell people not to worry about a night of poor sleep. Even a terrible night can be extremely valuable if managed well. In fact, get your handling right of that one night, and you'll make more progress with your insomnia recovery than with any number of good nights. It's how you cope when you make mistakes and when things *aren't* going well that will make you truly successful, not when things are easy.

It's the same with food. Learning a great mindset isn't just about eating well, it's about coping well when you *don't*. It's about dealing with those times when you mess up, overeat or eat the wrong thing.

Notice that self-rebuke *doesn't stop us doing the same thing again*. We are so busy beating the crap out of ourselves for eating the entire tub of ice cream that we don't even stop to log the fact that *eating this much ice cream doesn't feel good*. The moment that negative judgement kicks in, you've lost that connection. We are so tied up in self-contempt and regret we don't hear the voice that says *I don't want to do that anymore*. But get your handling of one episode of overeating right, and you could get such a powerful learning, you might never do it again.

So, give yourself permission to get it wrong. Let it be okay.

However, please don't use this as an excuse. Having permission to make mistakes is not carte blanche to eat until you are sick or free rein to complain mercilessly about your food and your body. But, *if* you overeat, *if* you eat something that doesn't agree with you, *if* you fail to do the Hero's Process, *if* you fall into negative self-talk, remember to treat it as a valuable learning experience and no harm will be done.

To do this, pay full and proper attention to the entire experience. Give as much attention to the experience as you can. Take a neutral, interested look at what has happened. Treat the whole experience as if you are a scientist doing an experiment, a neutral observer taking notes. There's nothing broken or wrong, just stuff to be noticed and loads to be learned.

For example, let's say you eat too much. More than that, you stuff yourself. Ask yourself:

Did you enjoy the whole experience? Be honest.

Do you feel good afterwards or bloated and rotten? Notice this.

Did you forget to do the Hero's Process? How did that affect your eating? Remember that.

What effect did not doing the Hero's Process have on your overall enjoyment of the experience? *Make a mental note.*

So, I'm not telling you to binge on ice cream. I'm telling you *if* you binge on ice cream, make sure you do the Hero's Process, pay full attention to the total experience, and get a valuable learning. We're looking for neutral observation, not self-flagellation. This way, even a full-blown binge can be a positive learning experience. When you let it all be okay, a binge isn't a disaster. It's information. *I ate a lot; I'm very full.* That's it. There is no negative story to be told.

If you allow the feeling of a binge to register, without beating yourself up for your gluttony, you can notice the way that bingeing makes you *feel*. You can then log in your memory how much you do or don't enjoy the entire experience. If you have ever eaten food that has made you throw up, you'll often find yourself unable to stomach this food again for many years. The experience has been logged; it has registered as unpleasant and not to be repeated. You can do exactly the same with overeating. As long as you give enough attention to the experience, use the Hero's Process and *let it be okay*. On some level, you'll log the knowledge that bingeing, overeating, or eating a certain food doesn't make you feel good. Proceed in this way, and you'll gain something amazing—the deep visceral understanding that ...

... you don't actually like overeating.

At that point, there will no longer be a compulsion to overeat. It won't seem remotely appealing when you properly register how bad it makes you feel. You won't want to overeat any more than you'll want to bang your head against a wall or poke yourself in the eye.

And all this, with no dieting. No restriction. No deprivation.

Just divine food freedom.

MAGIC ACTION STEP: GIVE YOURSELF PERMISSION TO PUT ON A LITTLE WEIGHT

Overeating is not the only subject where you're going to need to let things be okay. You also need to be okay with putting on a wee bit of weight in the early days.

Before you jump out of your skin or throw the book across the room, let me explain. I am categorically not saying you should *expect* to put on weight. I am saying you need to be okay with it, to *give yourself permission* to put on weight, at least at first.

This might be troublesome for you especially if you have recently come off a strict diet and have already lost a load of weight. The thought of ruining all your hard work may well appal you. If you are at your heaviest, the thought of hitting a new highest weight may horrify you even more. But if you *don't* allow these early fluctuations to be okay, you're likely to go off-plan and resort to another diet, imposing restrictions on what and how much you eat, ruining all your fine attempts to make genuine change.

You see, in order to create positive changes, all these new behaviours need to become a habit. During the first sixty days while the new habit is bedding in, your weight might move up or down. I know it's painful to accept the possibility of putting on more weight, but it's not like this hasn't happened before. How many times have you jumped on the scales in the past and found you'd put on a pound or two? And that was *despite* going on countless diets, *despite* doing your best to follow guidelines and *despite* trying exceedingly hard (and failing) to stay in control of your eating.

Can't you see? Restriction and dieting don't work the way you think they do. In fact, nothing you have done until now has worked. If it had, you wouldn't be here reading this book.

If you're still tempted by the few pounds of weight loss guaranteed by starting a new diet, remind yourself how it's always worked out in the past and how temporary that weight loss has always been.

Yes, having no restrictions is scary. But you're working towards something truly worthwhile. You're learning a new way of being around food, instilling a positive new habit, and effecting a real and lasting transformation. So, why does it matter if you were to put on a pound or two short term?

The reward will be worth it.

It might also help if you appreciate that weight loss alone is not a sign of success. After all, you could lose ten pounds, but if you haven't also changed the way you think around food, those pounds will probably pile straight back on in a matter of weeks.

On the other hand, if you *gain* a little weight in the short term but make huge changes in all the other areas we have talked about, it would count as a resounding success. It's those changes that will ultimately create *long-term, lasting* changes to your weight, your health and the entire way you experience the world. What we are doing here is infinitely more valuable and desirable than a few pounds of temporary weight loss. So let weight loss be a consequence, not a goal.

The actual goals of this book are:

1. feeling relaxed around food;

2. getting real satisfaction from the whole eating experience;

3. discovering the foods that are right for your body; and

4. being able to eat what you want, what is right for your body and in the right quantities without resorting to diets and third-party rules.

Weight loss is just a byproduct of all these other goodies. If we make it the primary focus, the supreme and solitary goal, this will interfere with all the other things we are trying to achieve.

So, give yourself time to find your groove. Let things settle in. Give your body and mind the chance to learn this new way of being, to make mistakes and learn from them, to play a wrong note and correct yourself and not to fall into self-recrimination or regret when this happens. Because there *will* be days when you end up eating more than your body wants. There will be days when you put on a pound or two. And that's fine because eating *more* than your body wants may be necessary for you to discover how much your body *actually* wants. So, forget the numbers on the scales. Forget the couple of pounds you may lose or gain in the short term. Forget the ticks in boxes and entries on charts.

But there's a problem ...

There's something that could make this aspect of 'letting everything be okay' terribly difficult:

Those bloody bathroom scales.

Getting on the scales each morning probably feels as insignificant and habitual as brushing your teeth. But it can have a devastating influence on all we are trying to achieve.

You see, if you get on your bathroom scales one morning and see a change in that number, either up or down, you won't be able to help but view it as a sign of progress or failure, and this will affect the way you *eat*.

If you get on the scales and you have *lost* weight, you may be less likely to eat what you want, because you'll be afraid of ruining all your hard work.

If you have *put on* weight, you may be tempted to nip that weight gain in the bud by restricting the amount you eat, starting calorie counting, or even bringing in a few of the old diet rules. You'll start thinking *I've put on a pound, I'd better be good today.* And by doing this, you'll fall back into the disordered thinking we are trying to overcome.

So, I'm going to make this easy. I'm going to suggest you ban yourself from stepping on the scales for at least sixty days. (Ideally, you would never weigh yourself again for the rest of your life!) I want you to have no idea how much you weigh—for your weight to be such a nonissue that you forget about it.

If sixty days sounds impossible, at least try not to jump on the scales until you reach a point of 'equilibrium'—a state of easy neutrality around food and your weight with intuition firmly back in control. Until then, *don't get on the scales!*

In fact, I'm going to recommend you go one stage further. Take your bathroom scales, put them in a bag, and take them down to your nearest charity shop (I think you Americans call them thrift stores). If there's no charity shop nearby, put them on Facebook Marketplace for a fiver. Failing that, chuck them in the bin.

I mean it. Get those guilt-inducing embodiments of arbitrariness out of your bathroom. If you can't bear to part with them, hide them in the attic or under your bed, or in some hard-to-reach cupboard where you can't easily get to them.

Because this is *not* a weight-loss plan. This is a getting-back-in-touch-with-your-body plan that will correct the disordered eating that may have been keeping you heavy.

To do this, we need to let *everything* be okay. And that includes overeating, weight gain, and eating the 'wrong' food. This is about being so okay with overeating, gaining weight and eating all the wrong foods that those things no longer happen.

Because it's the *not* letting everything be okay that opens the door to judgement, stories, guilt and shame.

It's the *not* letting everything be okay that clouds your intuition and keeps it hidden.

It's the *not* letting everything be okay that leads us to overeat in pursuit of happiness.

But when you *let everything be okay* and drop those negative judgements, your inner happiness bubbles up. And your innate intuition that *always makes the right food choices* is free to speak.

Chapter Twenty-Seven

I Get It Right and It's Okay

I remember the first bite of food I had after the insight that led to this book. My partner, Mike, and I were out with my granddaughter, Darcie, at a dinosaur-themed amusement park and we had stopped for lunch. Immediately prior to this, I had been starving myself on the paleo diet, eating nothing but tiny meals of meat and nonstarchy vegetables. And I was more than ready to try something properly tasty.

I ordered a cheese and ham toasted sandwich. During the months of paleo, I would not have been allowed any part of this sandwich, and I felt a noticeable trepidation about eating it. Was I about to blow all my hard work on paleo? What would the dairy in the cheese do to me? What about the wheat in the bread? Would it set off some terrible inflammation response? Would it start a binge?

(How ridiculous does this sound? Apprehension about eating a flipping sandwich!)

But I reminded myself, a cheese and ham sandwich was no longer forbidden. I had unconditional permission to eat it. In fact, I had unconditional permission to eat whatever I wanted later that day, that night and for the rest of my life.

As I bit into the sandwich, I reminded myself *You're allowed to eat this. You may eat anything. You may eat whatever you like for the rest of your life.*

And something odd happened. The sandwich didn't taste that good. It was too salty, too greasy. Halfway through, I closed my eyes and felt into the feelings in my body. I did a Mini Process and asked myself, 'Do I want more?' The answer was no; I wasn't notably hungry anymore, and the sandwich was doing nothing for me. I didn't see any point in eating the rest, given that I wasn't enjoying the experience. And so, I stopped. I left half the sandwich.

Shocker! Leaving half a sandwich? That would never have happened a year ago. My dissatisfaction with my meal would not have been enough to stop me finishing every bite.

What made the difference this time?

It's a simple question: do you want the damned sandwich? But all my life I had made it so, so difficult for myself. I was so used to employing reason and argument and externally imposed rules to answer that question. *Is it healthy, is it gluten free, is it keto, is it paleo, how much fat, how many carbs and calories does it have? Is it sourdough or wholemeal? It cost £15 so I'd better eat the whole thing.*

No wonder I felt out of control. I was always trying to rationalise my way to a decision about something utterly basic and instinctual.

But the act of allowing all food, any food whenever I liked, meant the mental tussle could stop. It relaxed the push and pull of thought, the confusing angsting over the simple act of eating. With all that mental noise out of the way and with that rational mind shut up for a moment, the quieter, truer, more intuitive magical voice could be heard. And it said, quite clearly and obviously, *I don't want to eat any more of this.*

So, the reason I 'got it right' is not because I left some food on my plate, or even because I ate less.

I got it right because I had given myself one hundred percent absolute, unconditional permission to eat.

I got it right because my decision to stop eating was based on intuition not intellect.

I didn't think my way to the answer. I didn't stop eating the cheese and ham sandwich because it contained too much saturated fat, its calorie content was too high, it wasn't in keeping with my daily macros, it wasn't gluten free, or because it wasn't paleo, keto, or WeightWatchers friendly. None of these rational, thought-based, externally validated reasons had any bearing on my stopping eating the sandwich. I stopped eating the sandwich because *I didn't want to eat any more.*

True, obvious, real, *right.*

Chapter Twenty-Eight

I Get It Wrong and It's Still Okay

As I write this, it's not even 9 a.m., and I've already eaten a pain au chocolate in a café. I bought it mindlessly, ate it mindlessly and realised about two-thirds through I wasn't enjoying it much. Today, I finished it anyway rather than stopping and leaving part of it on my plate. Now I'm sitting here with cold, hard pastry like a lump in my stomach. The coffee I've ordered has far too much milk added, giving it a slightly sticky, sour taste. But I'm drinking it anyway.

However, I'm not indulging in any self-recrimination. I resist the temptation to reach for my phone to check the calories in a pain au chocolate. The thought pops in, *you've had sugar for breakfast, so you should probably skip lunch and have a small dinner.* But I push it away.

I remind myself that it's fine to occasionally overeat. It's fine to eat something you don't enjoy now and again. As long as I *pay attention*, as long as I take the time to notice how I feel when I do this, as long as I don't give in to the stories my mind is telling me and beat myself up. No 'being bad', or 'ruining everything', or 'being a pig'. As long as I stay neutral, feel what's here, and grant myself access to the place beneath the story, I will learn from this. Because that part of me never lies; that part of me cannot ever get it wrong.

Somewhere, my body has logged this experience, the 'pains au chocolates aren't that nice and don't feel good in the tum' experience.

But this is not an experience of guilt or regret.

It's not an experience of ruining everything.

It's not an experience of being a fat pig who can't control her appetite and can't stick to anything.

This experience is information. It's data. It's information that I don't much like pains au chocolate and they don't feel nice in my tummy, particularly first thing in the morning.

I got this valuable information, this vital data, by looking *beneath* the stories about fat and carbs and sugar and being a fat, uncontrolled loser, to the simple fact of the raw feel of this moment. Where the wisdom, the intuition, the intelligence lies.

So, this experience of 'getting it wrong' (overeating a pain au chocolate) is an information-gathering, fact-finding experiment. Not a gluttonous mistake, but a valuable experience. Because next time I go into that coffee shop, I will probably skip the pain au chocolate!

So that was Strand 6. Let's just remind ourselves of the magic action steps for this strand.

1. GIVE YOURSELF PERMISSION TO MAKE MISTAKES
2. GIVE YOURSELF PERMISSION TO PUT ON A LITTLE WEIGHT

STRAND SEVEN

THE COMMITMENT TO HEROISM

Chapter Twenty-Nine

It Only Works if You Do It

That's actually most of the plan done. But there's something else I need to say. There's another thing needed to make this all work. This next part is not a different way to approach your weight issues, and there are no magic action steps specific to it. This strand is more to do with the way we approach the whole scheme itself.

What we need now is a commitment to follow these steps for a reasonable period of time. I know you're probably sick to death of commitment after so many years of strict dieting. However, what I'm suggesting is quite different to trying to stay below twelve hundred calories a day or vowing to give up sugar. On this plan, your food is your choice. The amount is your choice. All you must commit to is applying the steps for the next sixty days.

Here's all that laid out in detail:

1. Use the Hero's Process before and during eating to tune in to your innate wisdom.

2. Eat only what you truly want to eat and as much of it as you like.

3. Try an enormous variety of fresh and cooked foods and be open to experimentation.

4. Allow yourself to waste food where necessary.

5. Extract as much whole body and soul nourishment, enjoyment and satisfaction out of every meal, every forkful, and every bite by paying full attention to the experience of eating.

6. Refuse to complain about your body or your weight; start telling a new story and feel gratitude for your body.

7. Do not weigh yourself for at least sixty days.

So yes, this *is* a commitment. But I think you'll agree that compared to a standard calorie-controlled weight-loss diet, this will be easy.

Maybe you still don't feel this is the right time for you. Maybe you can't take the risk of trusting your ability to make the right decisions over food, and sixty whole days of your life is too long doing something so unconstrained. Perhaps you want to lose thirty pounds fast, and only a strict diet will deliver that.

However, think about this: You may well lose those thirty pounds, but they *will* come back. They always have, and given your history with dieting, chances are they always will. Your weight will go down, then it will go up. And you will be back on the rollercoaster, watching in despair as your weight creeps up and up, year on year as it always has after every other diet you've tried. You will remain at the mercy of the latest health fads, changing doctors' opinions, and every new bandwagon diet that promises the earth and doesn't deliver.

This pattern will continue until you take the brave step of doing something different, something courageous, something *heroic*.

The most courageous thing you can do regarding your body, food and diet is to start trusting yourself. Until you trust yourself, you have no option other than to trust others, and we all know where that leads.

Why not take the hero's way and start now? In a few months, you could look and feel like a whole different person.

Over the course of the next sixty days:

You will get used to eating only what you want.
You will no longer worry about the calories, carbs or fat in food.
You will get used to listening to your body and eating what food suits your body and soul.
You will get used to paying proper attention to the experience of eating.
You will get more satisfaction from your food and will find yourself stopping naturally when you've had enough.
You'll start to have a whole new respect for your amazing body.
You will realise at a deep, visceral level that it's okay to eat exactly what you want, as much as you want, without fear of putting on weight.

It won't be long before all these new behaviours will become second nature. The effort required will decline as everything becomes more instinctive. You'll get to the stage where doing the Hero's Process will take seconds, and you'll be doing it without having to stop and think. The sense of control will grow. The fear, the panic, the utter confusion around food will become a thing of the past. And you'll have found freedom, *true* freedom around food.

However, there's something important I need to say before we finish this strand. In fact, I can't emphasise this enough:

The plan only works if you do it.

I'm drawing attention to this stupidly obvious point because, bizarrely enough, it won't be easy to 'just do it'. It's not that anything I've suggested is unduly difficult, but because outside voices will question what you are doing, and doing that Hero's Process every time you eat is going to feel like a massive pain in the backside. Internal voices will try to make you rethink your commitment. The pull to do it the old way will be strong.

There will be:

The temptation to not bother with the Hero's Process before eating *just this once*
The temptation to weigh yourself *but only today*
The temptation to complain about your weight or your progress *this one time*
The temptation to choose the diet food *for this one meal*
The temptation to restrict your portion size *because this food is SO loaded with calories*
The temptation to ignore the Mini Process midmeal *because you're in a rush*
The temptation to eat in front of the TV *just because…*

These things will call to you, tempting you to fall back on old ways. The heroism comes in when you allow those temptations to be there without giving in to them. Each of these little temptations is another monster to overcome, another enemy to face. So, feel the strength of that pull to fall into unhelpful habits and don't give in. Buck your usual trend, resist that temptation to backslide into old ways. Face up to those little monsters and overcome them.

A commitment is necessary because most of the steps suggested here won't come easily until you've been doing them for a while. And until they feel easy, that commitment is what will keep you on track.

It's just sixty days of your life. Sixty days of *minor* effort and slight inconvenience to change your life forever.

And there's something quite important you need to know about this 'difficult' early stage. Feeling the initial discomfort is *necessary*. You don't get to avoid it. You must experience the discomfort, however minor, of doing something new and different.

The point is not to avoid discomfort.

The idea is to *feel* it. Feel that discomfort of doing something new until you no longer see it as something to be rid of.

The point is to experience it. All of it. When you accept the discomfort of following the plan *without wanting to drive it away or acting to fix it*, you'll experience the true power of this simple act.

This is how you slay the dragon. And it's the most unusual and transformative thing you can do.

While finishing this book, I happened across a YouTube video by neuroscientist Andrew Huberman talking about a part of the brain called the anterior midcingulate cortex.

Apparently, this part of the brain gets bigger when you tackle difficult tasks, and it shrinks when you avoid them. It's much bigger in those who are slim, and tiny in those who are very overweight. It's especially large in those who overcome real challenges. As it turns out, this part of the brain is also the seat of willpower, courage, tenacity and resilience.

This totally resonates with my experience. I have always noticed the more I step outside my comfort zone by doing the tough thing, the more fearless and happier I have become. All good things require something in return. And it seems to me that happy and successful people are often those who don't take the easy way out. They are those prepared to do the difficult thing in order to get what they want. Even my mastering of magic—that which makes everything *effortless*—required me to make considerable effort to get it. As I often say, you must make the effort to get to that effortless place.

The truth is, the more you do the difficult thing, the easier it gets to do difficult things. And this is not limited to big challenges like public speaking, starting a business, moving to a new country or leaving an abusive partner. I mean the small, mundane bothersome tasks too.

You may have thought it somewhat overdramatic to call this a hero's journey, but it's perfectly appropriate. The whole reason the concept of the hero's journey resonates so strongly with us is precisely because it shows up in our lives every single day.

What are the little battles you face every day? Try to see each challenge as a tiny clash with a dragon. A chance to do something different, to be a hero. Even if the struggle you overcome is making your bed when you don't want to, going to the gym when you're not in the mood, or following the Hero's Process when all you want to do is eat without thinking, you grow. Your world grows. (And I suspect your anterior midcingulate cortex grows too.) And what happens as a result? You become more courageous, more tenacious, more confident, and life gets happier, easier and less fearful.

If you can get used to sitting with discomfort and feeling it until it transforms, it's going to change your life in ways you can't even begin to imagine.

Every time you do the difficult thing, every time you choose not to run to safety and familiarity, every time you allow the discomfort to be there without trying to fix it, you win a small battle with a personal demon.

Whether it's facing a big fear or a minor irritation. Whether it's a craving for food or a craving for company. A yearning for the past or a desperate longing for *something else*. Face it. Feel it. Allow it. Do not run. Do not hide. Do not avert your gaze from the monster. Feel it and feel it all. Choose the hero's way, *always*.

Yes, I know it feels strange at first. It sounds wrong to move *into* discomfort rather than away. But, come on, this is *magic* we are doing.

You didn't expect magic to be the same old same old, did you? You didn't expect magic to feel routine and to align with everything else you've been told. Yes, magic is odd, it sounds wrong, it seems abnormal.

But everyone else is normal. Don't be normal. Be magic.

It's the unexpected, counterintuitive, oddness of magic that makes it so powerful. Because it takes bravery even to entertain the ideas of irrationality, of no scientific proof, and of magic itself. Even more than brave, it makes you *unusual*.

It also makes you one of my people.

Remember, at the end of the hero's journey, the protagonist comes home with the treasure? Well, now it's time to collect your reward.

And oh, the rewards of being one of us!

Sometimes, I feel I have been given the secret to life. I often feel I know something no one else does. Life is so, so simple. More than easy, beyond effortless. And hardly anyone knows.

All you have to do is feel, allow, push nothing away.

So now, the choice is yours. Are you going to fall back into the same old same old or are you going to turn in a different direction, an unexpected direction, a magical direction? *Are you willing to take the hero's path?* This path is not out into the world. The direction is into *yourself*, into your feelings, into the pain and suffering, and out the other side.

And the reward isn't just a lighter, slimmer, healthier body. It's also a calm, easygoing freedom around food you may never have experienced before.

But that's not all.

Your confidence will grow.
Your resilience will improve.
Your courage will reach a new level.
Your happiness levels will reach never-before-seen heights.
Your life will take on an exciting new momentum as you feel yourself actually growing into a *stronger, more powerful, more capable you.*

Weight loss? Weight loss is just the beginning!

***

You've now completed all seven strands of *Feasting on Magic*. And I hope you're excited to begin putting things into practise. I admit, that was a lot to get through. If you feel like you've already forgotten half of it, at the end of the book you'll find a cheat sheet that lists all the strands with a brief description of each you can refer to.

You can also download a printable version of the cheat sheet and an MP3 recording of the Hero's Process here https://www.becomingmagic.com/feasting-resources/

However, we're not done yet. I've added three great bonus sections. Turn to those now. They are a lot of fun!

THE BONUSES

Bonus 1: Superpowering Your Weight Loss With Fasting

I can talk all day about the importance of contacting your intuition, and trusting yourself, and having freedom around food all day long. But we both know that what you're here for is weight loss.

Yes, of course, you want to feel more relaxed around food. Of course, you want to enjoy your food without guilt. Of course, you want an alternative to dieting. But if what you want most of all is to be thinner, keep reading and open yourself up to possibly the healthiest, most spiritual, and most effective way to achieve that.

The sixty-day plan I've presented *will* help you lose weight, but it might take longer than you'd like. For some of you, the desire to be smaller as soon as possible is stronger than the desire for permanent, lasting change. Even after all I've said about the pitfalls of dieting, you may still be tempted to try that new diet you heard about so you can drop a few pounds as quickly as possible.

Wouldn't it be great if there were a way you could get in touch with your intuition and develop a healthy relationship with food, while also losing weight at a satisfying rate?

There is. I'm talking about *intermittent fasting*.

- *But hang on one minute! Fasting? Aren't we supposed to eat whatever we want? Aren't we supposed to listen to our intuition? Doesn't fasting blatantly ignore our natural, healthy hunger cues by basically starving ourselves and drowning out that inner intuition to eat?*

Strangely enough, fasting turns out to be a remarkably helpful addition to this plan. It fits perfectly because, as we've discussed, you can eat whatever you want in whatever quantities you want. The sole restriction is time. You don't get to eat *when* you want.

So, you can have what you want and as much as you want. You just can't necessarily have it *now*. You *can* have it later. This means a well-managed fast once or twice a week could give you the nirvana you are looking for because you get to lose weight at a steady rate with no restrictions on food type or quantity.

But that's not all. I've discovered there's so much more to fasting than simply an easy way to lose weight.

For a start, my experience of regular fasting has left me with something astonishingly valuable. It's given me *a different relationship with hunger itself*. In the developed world, most of us rarely experience true hunger. At least, not for very long. Food is everywhere. If we live in a city, we can step outside our front door and find a dozen places offering food within a couple of minutes. Our cupboards and fridges are full. We have so much we use freezers to store the excess. And if we have little food in the house, we can pick up the phone and have almost any food delivered within an hour. When we're hungry, we eat. For many of us, then, we never experience hunger unless we're on a diet. This can mean that the sensation of hunger is associated with deprivation, restriction and misery.

But fasting is different. When fasting, we *choose* to go without food rather than being deprived of it. This means we get the chance to experience the sensation of hunger intimately without a negative emotional charge. In this way, we can learn much about it. For example, we discover that hunger comes and goes and that some days we are hungrier than others. I've done sixteen-hour fasts where I felt hungrier than I did on a forty-eight-hour fast. I've had days when I've woken up famished and others when I've forgotten to eat until dinner time.

But most interestingly, we discover that hunger does not increase much with time. It doesn't ramp up hour by hour and day by day. Whether you've fasted for fourteen hours or three days, the intensity of your hunger is nearly the same. So, a three-day fast may be more boring than a twenty-four-hour fast. But other than that, it's not any more difficult or unpleasant.

And finally, we learn the difference between genuine hunger and craving. We see that genuine hunger is about a need for food, whereas craving is often about a need for something else—happiness, belonging, love or entertainment. We also learn genuine hunger is far easier to resist than craving.

We might imagine that after twenty hours of no food, we will be so ravenous we will stuff our faces the moment we sit down to eat and ruin all our efforts. But this is not what happens. Anyone who has tried intermittent fasting will have noticed this. After a long fast, we often find ourselves full and satisfied with far less food than usual.

Overall, we form a different relationship with this mysterious sensation. We learn that hunger is not an alarm bell, not a danger siren, not an action call to *eat, eat, eat NOW!* And so, we become less afraid of it and feel less need to respond instantly with food. We get to feel hunger in its pure state for possibly the first time, without any story that it's wrong or must be fixed. It's a rather strange but rather interesting experience and not nearly as unpleasant as we previously assumed.

If you're into the science, you'll be interested to learn that fasting for periods of at least sixteen hours may also be incredibly good for you. It's after about sixteen to twenty hours of fasting that *autophagy* kicks in. Autophagy is the body's own natural cleansing system—a process of literally burning up the dodgy and mutated cells that are bumbling around our bodies. If those dodgy cells are left to float about, some of them can end up turning into cancer. Autophagy means those cells are eaten up by the body and used as energy before they can wreak their horrible damage. This means you can get massive health benefits *without changing a thing about what you eat*.

I like the sound of autophagy. Instinctively, it makes sense to me. When fasting, I never say 'I'm hungry'. I always say 'I'm healing', because I've come to associate the sensation of hunger with the idea of autophagy. I can't help but imagine my body hoovering up stray cancer cells and other nasties. This takes a lot of the sting out of the hunger.

Still, I know better than to blindly accept the words of others. So I don't. I like the idea of autophagy and I hope it's true. But it's not the main reason I fast. I fast because I like the way fasting makes me feel. If it made me feel rotten, I wouldn't do it. Simple as that.

Since starting experiments with fasting, I've discovered twenty-four-hour fasts (e.g., from after dinner at 7 p.m. to 7 p.m. the next evening) to be quite easy. Fasts of up to about fifty hours make me feel sharp, energetic and awake. I have fasted for as long as five days, but I haven't felt good. Longer fasts appear to weaken me, making my thinking fuzzy and affecting my decision-making. I don't feel right on a very long fast, so I don't do them. But this is just me. Your mileage may well vary. I took to fasting like a duck to water partly because I almost never feel hungry in the mornings. Incidentally, did you know that 'Breakfast is the most important meal of the day' is nothing but a marketing message made up by a cereal company? I find it quite worrying that children now accept that there is something wrong if they go to school on an empty stomach. Even as a child, I almost never ate breakfast before school because I found the prospect of eating first thing in the morning quite nauseating. I feel much sharper and my gym workouts are easier when I skip breakfast. But my mother, for instance, wouldn't dream of skipping breakfast, being unable to function without it. For her, skipping dinner is easier than going without breakfast. I love my twenty-four-hour fasts, but my partner, Mike, prefers longer fasts of two to three days at a time rather than several shorter ones. The point here is not to emulate my behaviour or blindly follow someone else's advice. I'm suggesting you experiment with fasting to find out what works for you.

HOW TO GET STARTED WITH FASTING

Starting fasting can be as simple as deciding to skip breakfast. If you finished your last meal of the day by 7 p.m. and ate nothing until 11 a.m. the next day, this would represent a sixteen-hour fast, which is a great place to start. If you're used to snacking in the evening and eating a big breakfast, this sixteen-hour fast could result in a pretty dramatic reduction in your size and weight. You may find even a sixteen-hour fast difficult at first. But I promise you, in time, your 'fasting muscle' will strengthen, and you'll find yourself quite ready to go for longer periods. Anything seems impossible, until you do it.

If you're new to fasting, I'm going to suggest that you start with:

1. A sixteen-hour fast each day. That's no food at all, not even a snack, between the hours of 7 p.m. and 11 a.m. or 6 p.m. and 10 a.m.

2. A twenty-four-hour fast is also known as 'one meal a day'. To do this, eat a standard evening meal and then have no food at all, not even a snack, until dinner time on the following day.

I especially like these twenty-four-hour fasts. I find my mind is sharp as a tack all day, I have tons of energy and I *really* enjoy my evening meal. The weight loss is the cherry on the cake. And what's most pleasing is that this weight seems to stay off rather than come piling back the moment you eat.

During fasting hours, you may drink water and black coffee only. No juice. No low-calorie drinks. Opinions vary over whether it's okay to drink teas, and even to add a little cream or full-fat milk to your coffee. I add a little milk to my one morning coffee, and everything still seems to work fine. Even Jason Fung, who is a huge proponent of intermittent fasting, says it's better to do a fast with a little cream in your coffee than not to fast at all.

This level of fasting should be doable for anyone without a medical condition. Obviously, if you have a known reason you shouldn't limit your eating in this way, you shouldn't fast. If in doubt, you must **always** consult your doctor.

WHAT ABOUT LONGER FASTS?

If you know you're fit and healthy, you might like to do some research into longer fasts of forty-eight hours or more. I'm not advising this, because I know nothing of your situation or medical history. I'm going to *recommend* fasting for no more than twenty-four hours because I'm neither a doctor nor a dietitian, and I don't want to take the risk of telling you to do something that might not be right for you. What I will do, is to tell you *my* experience with longer fasts.

Here's what I've discovered: Longer fasts aren't just great for weight loss, they also have some transformative effects on our well-being. For one, we come to see how much of our day is taken up with activities related to food. Whether it's thinking about what to eat, shopping for food, preparing it, cooking it, eating it or talking about what we just ate, food uses up a lot of our day. When all those activities are suddenly gone, we notice what all that activity and busyness was covering up. You find that 'stuff comes up'. Sometimes this is in the form of memories or emotions you have been hiding for years. You might experience deep grief, shame or a sense of loss. But this is not a negative thing. Discovering these hidden emotions signals immense catharsis. By applying the Hero's Process to all these emotions by feeling deeply into them, they will release their hold on you.

When this deep-seated, long-hidden pain comes up and out, the relief and transformation can be spectacular. World-changing insights occur. Deep, lifelong problems, struggles and issues leave you. And when that sort of pain is gone, it's gone for good. Little wonder that so many of the world's great religions include fasting as part of their spiritual practice.

I have experienced bliss, ecstasy, moments of extraordinary understanding and even mystical visions while fasting. I've gone through the excruciating boredom of no food and found truly incredible truths on the other side. I've learned so much, all because I didn't eat for a while!

What I appreciate most about fasting is that it is so flexible. You don't need to do it every day. You can choose the days you wish to fast and the days you don't. This means fasting fits in with almost any lifestyle and doesn't interfere with most social events. You could not eat after 6 p.m., skip breakfast and lunch the next day and go out to dinner that evening, eating whatever you like, and you'd still have managed a twenty-four-hour fast! That makes it close to weight-loss nirvana in my book.

This is not a long section because there's not much you need to know about fasting other than 'don't eat for a bit'. It's true, there are often minor unwanted side effects such as headaches, lethargy and mood changes. But these can often be relieved with a good electrolyte supplement. Just search Amazon for 'electrolytes for fasting'. You'll also find loads of great books written on the subject of fasting. So do some research if you want to. Talk to your doctor if you want some reassurance. Or just decide one day not to eat for a bit.

That's all fasting is.

Bonus 2: Help! I'm Going To Binge!

This bonus section is specifically about *bingeing*—that most uncontrolled, frantic form of overeating. I urge you to read this section carefully, even if bingeing has never been a problem for you. Seeing how the plan applies to bingeing is a great way to illustrate the whole program in action, and everyone should find the material here hugely helpful. So do read on, there's gold in the following pages.

BINGE NIGHT THE OLD WAY

It's the day from hell. There was that negative appraisal at work, and your boss is concerned about your performance. A huge, unexpected bill has come in, and you have no money to pay it. It's Friday, and you're on your own with no fun plans for the weekend to look forward to. Your commute home from work took ages. You're starving and there's nothing in the fridge. And, to add insult to injury, you've scrolled through Facebook and seen a photo of your ex-husband on holiday with his gorgeous new wife. You're now utterly wretched.

All you want to do is order a fifteen-inch pizza and a tub of Häagen-Dazs (or whatever your chosen comfort food would be) and eat yourself into a stupor. The idea of eating tons of something delicious feels utterly irresistible. All you can think about is drowning in food. The decision is made; the only thing that can make this awful day better is a feast in front of the TV.

The pizza arrives, and you sit on your sofa, remote control on one side, pizza box on the other, to begin your feast. You turn on a nice rom com or crime drama to increase the pleasure.

As you take the first bite, a wave of happiness rushes up through you. The pizza is delicious, all you had hoped for. The next bite is equally good. You eat rapidly, mindlessly, hardly chewing, seemingly filling the unhappiness with food. Little attention is given to the experience of eating or even to the food itself. You simply stuff the food down in a desperate, panicky and almost frenzied mission to feel better.

Before long the guilt and regret start to kick in.

You're eating too much. Stop now. Are you seriously going to take another slice of pizza? You've already had four. Why are you being such a pig? Why can't you control yourself?

But you don't stop. If you stop eating, you will have to face up to what you have done. In order to soothe those feelings and silence the uncomfortable thoughts, you just eat more. The feelings you are now trying to block include guilt and shame about the binge itself.

As the binge goes on, the guilty feelings intensify. This meal now has nothing to do with hunger or even with wanting food. You're in a vicious circle, trying to counter revulsion, guilt and shame from eating so much *by eating even more.*

Now you're in binge hell.

All this guilt and emotional stress blinds you to your natural wisdom, blocking access to the normal, healthy intuitions that tell you when you've had enough. You stop only when you're stuffed to the neck, dejected and disgusted with yourself. And now you're so full, you can't even eat to make yourself feel better.

What a way to start your weekend.

BINGE NIGHT THE HERO'S WAY

I'm now going to show you a calm approach to navigating the various stages of a binge, avoiding all the panic, fear and loss of control. And again, even if you're not prone to bingeing, do read on. You will still find what I say here extremely helpful.

Let's say you're in a great place now. You've made your commitment to the eating plan in this book, and for a couple of weeks, you've been choosing the food your body really wants. You are eating it mindfully and paying full attention to the experience. You've found a taste for new and healthy foods. You've let go of much of the guilt and self-recrimination around food and have even thrown away your bathroom scales. Your clothes are slightly looser, and you feel better within yourself. You are optimistic and positive about the future, and all seems rosy.

Then ... a bad day comes along.

It's the day from hell. There was that negative appraisal at work, and your boss is concerned about your performance. A huge, unexpected bill has come in, and you have no money to pay. It's Friday, and you're on your own with no fun plans for the weekend to look forward to. Your commute home from work took ages. You're starving and there's nothing in the fridge. And, to add insult to injury, you've scrolled through Facebook and seen a photo of your ex-husband on holiday with his gorgeous new wife. You're now utterly wretched.

All you want to do is order a fifteen-inch pizza and a tub of Häagen-Dazs (or whatever your chosen comfort food would be) and eat yourself into a stupor. The idea of eating tons of something delicious feels utterly irresistible. All you can think about is drowning in food. The decision is made; the only thing that can make this awful day better is a feast in front of the TV.

So, what's changed now that you're taking the Hero's way? How will you tackle this situation differently?

First, *give yourself full permission to eat whatever it is you really want*. Remember, there must be no restrictions on food, either in choice or amount. Restriction will set up another level of resistance and bad feeling, pushing you to eat even more. So right from the start, tell yourself no food is off-limits. You can eat whatever you want without guilt. This is extremely important, and you should not reject it no matter how counterintuitive it feels. If tonight you want to eat pizza and ice cream, then eat pizza and ice cream. You are allowed to have Chinese takeaway. You are allowed fish and chips. You are even allowed to eat nothing but chocolate if that's honestly what you want.

Next, remind yourself there will be no diet starting Monday. There will be no diet ever again for the rest of your life. You're able to eat pizza whenever you want. So you don't need to eat it all now if you don't want to. This removes that urge to eat everything in sight because there's another diet starting on Monday.

Sometimes, just giving yourself these permissions is enough to change everything. When you slow down, take a breath and give yourself calm permission to eat pizza and ice cream, *now and forever*, you may discover that pizza and ice cream are not actually what you want.

But let's suppose you *do* still want them. The next step is to give yourself full permission to eat as much as you want. This is not carte blanche to eat yourself into oblivion. This is not permission to binge. It's not even permission to overeat. It's permission to eat *as much as you want*. And I think we can all agree that bingeing or eating to the point of discomfort is not about eating as much as you want. Overeating, almost by definition, is about eating *far more* than you want. It's about eating *even when you don't want to.*

By giving yourself permission to eat what you want and in whatever quantities, you can begin communicating with the part of you that wants, that needs, that *knows* what you actually want. Denial, restriction, judgement and misplaced morality are sure ways to cut the connection to your inner wisdom. So, give yourself a fighting chance of finding your own magical food wisdom—the wisdom that doesn't require restriction or rules, the wisdom that already knows what's right.

Back to your imminent binge. How do you get in touch with this uncorrupted, knowing part of you *right now*?

Simple. You do the Hero's Process.

You may eat as much as you want of whatever you want, but *only* if you first carry out the process. This is the one restriction you must respect. Underneath all the stories and judgements and food rules, under the misunderstood craving—the nagging voices that say 'this food will make you happy'—is a knowing voice, a crystal-clear sense of wanting in this moment. And when you get in touch with the basic, simple desire in this moment, you will find something amazing ...

... no compulsion to binge, no lack of control, not even any desire to overeat.

Instead, you find one of two things:

a simple desire for this particular food at this particular moment,

or

no desire for this particular food at this particular moment.

So do the Hero's Process. Reach the true wisdom, the authentic desire for food that sits beneath. This wisdom will never encourage you to overeat. It will never fat shame you, never berate you for getting it wrong. Never tell you the answer to your bad mood is to eat more.

Without the process, *without* permission to eat, *without* making the effort to do something a wee bit different:

In an hour, you'll be in binge hell.

In two hours, you'll be sick, bloated and regretful.

And you'll have learned *nothing*. So do the process. Avoid that hell. Avoid the diet starting Monday. Avoid the creep, creep up of your weight. Avoid the breathlessness, the lack of energy, the low self-esteem.

Back to our miserable Friday night.

We start the Hero's Process on whatever emotional discomfort is foremost. This evening, you know you're definitely hungry. But you also feel hurt, rejection, shame, fear of missing out and perhaps jealousy from seeing your ex with a new partner. You may be angry about what happened at work. You may also feel bored, irritated and in need of entertainment, lonely at the prospect of a weekend alone. You may not even know quite what you feel, you only know you want to feel better than *this*.

Don't worry about correctly identifying exactly what you feel. It's not remotely important to name your feelings.

All you need to do is use the Hero's Process to feel the discomfort of whatever feeling is there until something shifts.

Close your eyes and feel. Let it all be there.

Say an internal *yes* to the sensation.

Feel it. And then a little more. And if you can, plunge deeply into the depths of that emotion and give yourself over to feeling the entirety of it.

Having felt deeply into the emotion that is uppermost in your experience, things should feel quite different. Some of the discomfort may still be there, but it will have lessened or changed.

So, the painful feelings motivating you to eat have eased off. The next step is to feel into the *craving itself*. (If there's anything left of it!)

Assuming you still have a craving, bring up that desire for pizza and ice cream. Where is that craving? Is it in your mouth, your tummy?

This bit is important.

Allow yourself to feel the craving *as craving*, making no attempt to avoid it, explain it or drive it out. Allow it to be there in all its intensity. Let yourself fall right into its toe-curling, stomach-twisting depths. Feel the craving until it changes. Don't push it away. Within seconds or minutes, the craving will either decrease or change into something else.

If a change in feeling doesn't happen straight away, repeat the process two to three times until something shifts.

Once that shift has happened—once you feel calmer, more peaceful, freer, happier, it's time to ask yourself:

What do I really want?

You may be astonished to discover that your previous craving for pizza and ice cream has transformed into a desire for a different food. You might now fancy something a little more wholesome or just a snack.

You may even discover you don't want food anymore. Instead, what you want is a chat with a friend or an early night with a book.

But if not, no worries. If all you are left with at this point is genuine, healthy physical hunger and a genuine desire for the pizza, great! You can now eat without worry, without guilt, without shame.

This is the beauty of doing the Hero's Process; it doesn't forbid you from eating. If you still want the pizza after doing the process, it doesn't mean you've failed. *It means you've genuinely discovered what you really want to eat.*

So go ahead. You now have full permission to eat the pizza and ice cream.

You are not eating it to blot out bad feelings; you're eating it because it's what you truly want to eat. And the difference is massive. Because now there's no guilt or shame. There's no need to stuff it down without thinking or tasting. Remember, *you're allowed to eat this*. So, enjoy it! Eat the pizza and ice cream slowly and with awareness of its taste. Pay attention to the way the food makes you feel. Savour each delicious morsel, extracting every drop of pleasure from each mouthful. *You're allowed this stuff, remember?*

Every few minutes, stop and check whether the food is still having the desired effect. Stop, put your knife and fork down and quickly tune in to your body again. Do a Mini Process for sixty seconds to get back in touch with your pure, natural wanting.

Then return to enjoying your meal.

There's no need to rush. Why waste the experience by eating it so fast you don't even taste it? Savour that pizza, enjoy the hell out of that ice cream. *Really* enjoy it.

And when you've stopped enjoying it, *stop eating it.*

You'll be amazed to discover that you effortlessly stop eating much sooner than usual, and far short of a full-blown binge.

The result is this: Instead of binge hell, you are left with a nice, comfortable full tummy. You've had a delicious Friday night meal, with no bloat or discomfort, guilt or shame. You've also gone through a massive learning experience and made the likelihood of another binge far less likely in the future.

In addition, the painful emotion that led you to eat in the first place has weakened or even disappeared. Rather than being depressed and lonely, you're now positive and optimistic about the coming weekend.

Isn't that worth a little effort? Isn't that worth a sixty-day commitment to a few behaviour changes?

Bonus 3: For Advanced Magicians

Adventure tales have a way of changing direction right at the end. Good stories have a development or two we didn't see coming. So here, at the end of the book, I offer you the final twist.

Get ready, we're going *full magic*.

As you already know, I'm not a dietitian, a weight-loss specialist or even an intuitive-eating coach. I'm a teacher of magic. And I've included this final, rather bizarre section as a nod to those of you who have been following me for some time and who are ready for a more advanced, slightly more magical explanation of what's going on.

When I ran the course that inspired this book, some participants were strangely quiet about this section. And I warn you now, what I'm about to say is pretty deep, it's not easy to understand, and it's probably not for beginners to magic. If you read what follows and don't understand a single bloody word, don't worry about it. The plan as it stands will work perfectly well.

I've introduced the Hero's Process as a means of getting in touch with your intuition about food. But the truth is, it's so much more than that. The process is essentially a way of letting *feelings* be okay, no matter how uncomfortable they are. This allows you to drop into that calm, peaceful, intuitive place.

I've often called this calm place of profound nonjudgement at the heart of every moment *the receiving state*. And the reason I call it a receiving state is that when you hang out here, you tend to receive things you want. And these things are not confined to good feelings and a sense of ease or peace. The receiving state will give you *real physical things*, including *the body you want*.

Yes, I mean that.

From the very beginning of my working with magic, I've noticed this phenomenon: When I stop grasping and yearning for something, surrender attachment to the outcome, let everything be profoundly okay, and enter the receiving state, *good things come to me*. Money, luck, opportunities, all the right people and all the right circumstances, wild synchronicities and serendipities. But it's only been in the last couple of years that I have got some understanding of what is going on, how and why it works. I'll give you a brief explanation. But I warn you, you may need to make a mental quantum leap in order to grasp what I'm saying here. It's not extraordinarily complicated, but it is weird.

In no way should you try to understand what I'm about to say rationally. You won't be able to. Instead, see if something resonates, that it makes sense even though you can't explain why. Try to feel into this rather than to understand.

The imperfection you see in your body, the sense of it being wrong and any idea that it needs to change are stories, concepts, a creation of your own beliefs. If your body doesn't look the way you want, it is because you're judging it as not right. You literally create a not okay situation by the act of judging it as not okay.

When you tell a story of being overweight, being slim or of anything at all, you literally make that true with the story you tell and the beliefs you hold.

This maybe sounds a bit like the law of attraction, but what I'm saying is different. Telling a story doesn't cause that situation to manifest. The story *is* the manifestation.

The belief doesn't affect what you experience. The belief *is* what you experience. The wrongness doesn't cause the negative judgement. The wrongness *is* the negative judgement. Judgement is the only place wrongness can exist.

If you told a story that you are slim, that you never struggled with weight and that you can eat what you want and never gain weight, and *truly believed it*, that's exactly what you'd experience.

Take a look at some naturally slim people. Not those with an eating disorder or those who lost weight after extreme dieting. I mean *naturally* slim. Naturally thin people eat whatever the hell they like. And they seem able to eat way more than us without gaining an ounce. They may believe *I have a fast metabolism* or *I've always been the same weight*. They may even believe (and I've heard this a lot from thin people) *I can't put weight on no matter what I eat.*

It's the belief that does it. The belief dictates the thoughts, dictates the actions, dictates the way they see their bodies *and their size and shape too*.

Now we can see yet another reason diets don't work. When you go on a diet, you tell the story with your words, thoughts and deeds that *there's something wrong with you, something not okay*. In practice, the act of going on a diet reinforces the belief that you are overweight. And as long as you believe you're overweight, that's exactly what you'll experience.

So, we end up with a horrible paradox. Doing things to try to lose weight is reinforcing the belief that you need to lose weight.

But what this means, in a sneaky twist of irony, is that everything we've talked about in this plan so far is, in a sense, *making things worse*. In following this program, you are essentially telling the story *I need to lose weight. I can't control my eating. I have a problem. I'm too fat. This needs to change.*

Even by picking up this book in the first place, you reinforced the belief that you need to be changed, effectively telling the story that there is something wrong with you. And while you continue to believe that there is something wrong with you, your body or your weight, that's exactly what you will experience. It may sound like impossible pie-in-the-sky nonsense, but if you could be truly okay with the body you have, *you would get the body you want.*

So, if I wanted to give you a streamlined, more accurate and truthful set of instructions, it would be this:

1. Eat one hundred percent freely for the rest of your life.

2. Know that your perfect body is already here.

3. Believe that you won't put on weight by eating.

4. Accept that the state of affairs you want so much is already here now.

5. Notice that what's standing in the way of what you want is your belief that it isn't already here.

6. Realise the less you judge this moment as lacking, the less you find it to be lacking. When you no longer lack, you *have*.

7. Stop believing there's something wrong with you, and you'll realise there never was.

That's what I want to tell you. Because that's the actual truth.

- *But how do I go about believing I have a perfect body, when I clearly don't. How do I go about believing I'm slim when I'm not? How do I accept that everything is okay when I don't think it is?*

Well, I'm not pretending this is easy. Simple, yes. Straightforward also. But no matter how many times I say it, or how I phrase it, 'letting everything be okay' is not always an easy piece of advice to follow and realising *everything is essentially perfect* is even harder. Hence, my books and programs, and my Academy of Magic with all its lessons and workshops and constant reinforcement of this simple, simple truth. Because even when the truth is simple, the implementation often isn't.

I've made this entire program, with all its bells and whistles, with all its steps and instructions for one reason: it's all been a sort of trick, a ruse, an attempt to poke insights out of you, to nudge those beliefs along.

So, until it's clear to you that you already *have* the perfect body, do absolutely follow the plan as laid out here. Take the practical steps and keep doing them. They are designed carefully to inspire the insights you need.

But more than any of that, keep doing the Hero's Process.

Keep feeling your feelings whenever and wherever you can.

Do this, and I promise you changes will occur. Your realisation will grow. Your understanding will transform. Insights will come to you. Things will begin to click.

And eventually you'll see the truth, plain as day:

You don't need to change. You never needed to change. You're already perfect.

But that's not all.

We *think* we want a 'perfect body'. We *think* we want to be able to eat what we want and not gain weight. We *think* we want to overcome our weight problems.

But in truth, that's not what we want. All we want is to be happy. We hanker after weight loss and the perfect body because we think those things will give us the happiness we seek. But because we spend our whole lives trying to find happiness in the wrong place and the wrong things, we never find what we are looking for. Thanks to that, the wanting continues, and the search lasts a lifetime.

So how *do* we find what we are looking for?

Many years ago, in one of my early books on magic, I wrote, 'wanting is the opposite of having'. This is true because wanting, by its nature, points away from here and now.

When we stop wanting, we stop looking away. We automatically find ourselves 'here', and consequently move closer to the true source of all we are looking for.

Remember, from Strand 4, happiness is not achieved or created through the act of eating, getting a thinner body or by doing things we love. Neither does it just appear. It is revealed.

When wanting stops, happiness remains.

The reason you don't feel it every moment of the day is because you believe the thoughts that tell you something is still wrong, that this moment is not okay. These thoughts tell you to *want things*. They direct you to look in the wrong place, out into the world, for something that isn't *this*.

But all along, happiness was already here and now.

Indeed, you could almost say happiness *is* the here and now.

You can't see it though because something is covering it up. What's hiding it is the wanting for this moment to be different. It's the sense of *I want something. I need something.*

But that wanting does not need to be sated. The discomfort does not have to be alleviated. The feeling does not have to be fixed. All we need to do is allow that feeling of lack to be present, to feel it fully without trying to fill it or repair it with food or distraction or drugs or by a different number on the scales. The craving, discomfort and all the other feelings *need to be felt*.

So 'feeling your feelings' doesn't pertain only to your relationship to food or eating or any other form of addiction. It applies to all of life. Use the process and keep using it with all uncomfortable feelings. The results will be automatic, and they will be incredible.

It turns out this book is about so much more than weight loss, food freedom or body confidence. The straightforward act of paying attention to how your body feels in any moment is a tool for *so* much more. The simple feel of your own body is your gateway to the divine and following the Hero's Process is an act of magic in itself.

If you're new to my work, my dearest wish would be that this book may be your 'in' to magic—an entryway, a portal to the magical you. This means your weight problem or your money problem could well turn out to be your greatest gift. It could be *the* thing that puts you in touch with your inner magical wisdom in a deeper and clearer way than ever before. In time, you may even end up grateful you had a weight problem in the first place. Your weight problem could end up being your launching pad to the fulfilment of all your dreams.

And all you have to do is *feel*.

You'll soon discover that feeling through *any* wanting results in that wanting dropping away. And if you exercise the process thoroughly, you may even find something rather fabulous. You may find yourself in a remarkable state where *you don't want anything at all*. If so, congratulations, you've received another treasure. You've found the perfect now. The place of peace and happiness at the heart of all of us. Here, you find there's no need to search for more or different. You discover, to your astonishment, that the present moment was perfect all along.

When you see the perfection of this moment, you can *finally* drop the exhausting and futile struggle to mend yourself, sort your life, and change what's already here. When you allow *everything* to be okay, even the way you feel right at this moment ...

... that's when you receive the secret special gold medal super-duper superhero's prize ...

... Home. Peace. Rest. Love.

You find The Kingdom of God.

Everything you've been looking for your whole life.

So, take this hero's path, find the place you've spent a lifetime looking for, and come home with the gold.

Feasting On Magic Cheat Sheet

Visit https://www.becomingmagic.com/feasting-resources/ to get this as a downloadable one-page PDF along with an MP3 of the Hero's Process.

Strand 1: NO RESTRICTIONS, NO RULES, NO DIETS

We have been listening to external advice for so long, we have developed learned helplessness around food. Because diets impose rules and restriction, they cannot work. Diets suppress our own intuition, stop us getting full body and soul satisfaction from our food, leading us to overeat. To make lifelong changes we must: 1) get full satisfaction from food, and 2) learn to consult our intuition. To achieve this, there should be no restrictions on our food either in terms of type or quantity.

MAGIC ACTION STEP: Eat *whatever* you want.
MAGIC ACTION STEP: Eat *as much* as you want.

And to ensure we don't overeat, we must combine the advice of this strand with the rest of the plan.

Strand 2: BEHAVIOURAL TRICKS

If we don't get full satisfaction from a meal, we will tend to overeat. We can get full satisfaction out of every meal by making a few simple behavioural changes. Eat at a table, serve yourself from dishes, put your cutlery down between bites and eat slowly. You will get more satisfaction from your experience and will naturally eat less without restriction. If food is not fully enjoyed, it is wasted whether you eat it or not. By permitting yourself to waste food now, you will save yourself wasting tons in the future.

MAGIC ACTION STEP: Pay more attention to the experience of eating.
MAGIC ACTION STEP: Allow yourself to waste food.

Strand 3: CHANGING UNWANTED BELIEFS

When we negatively judge ourselves, our food and our bodies, this leads to self-reproach and body shame. This blocks our intuition and mars the experience of eating with guilt and humiliation. Without full satisfaction, we overeat again. Given the power of placebo, it must be the case that the beliefs we hold affect the shape and size of our bodies and even the nutritional effects of our food. There are three ways we can effectively change these beliefs.

MAGIC ACTION STEP: Tell the story that you would like to be true about your body, your weight and your food.
MAGIC ACTION STEP: Stop complaining about your body, your weight and your food.
MAGIC ACTION STEP: Learn to love your body by standing naked in front of a mirror and being grateful for the body you have.

Remember, the only way to get the body you want is to be fully accepting of the one you have now.

Strand 4: FINDING INTUITION

Overeating is simply one version of the universal search for happiness. We will never find that happiness in food because that's not where it comes from. Happiness comes from within us. It is the feeling that remains when the wanting *stops*. This means what we crave is actually the end of craving. By feeling deeply into the craving for food, without submitting to it, we find an honest, obvious wanting to eat or not eat. This is the seat of intuition about food. This is what I call pure wanting.

MAGIC ACTION STEP: Use the Hero's Process to feel deeply into and through deeply uncomfortable feelings.
MAGIC ACTION STEP: Use the Hero's Process on a strong urge or craving to eat.
MAGIC ACTION STEP: Use the Mini Process partway through a meal to check if you've had enough and prevent overeating.

IMPORTANT: We don't use the process to restrict our eating; we use it to discover whether we want to eat at all.

Strand 5: DISCOVER YOUR INNER NUTRITION EXPERT

A human being must be capable of making nutritionally correct food choices. Somewhere deep inside is the ability to choose food that is right for our bodies *and* our souls. By experimenting with lots of new foods and unfamiliar foods, and by paying attention to the way a food makes you feel during and after eating it, you will discover what foods are perfectly right for you.

MAGIC ACTION STEP: Experiment with lots of new and unfamiliar foods.
MAGIC ACTION STEP: Use the Hero's Process to discover your personal nutrition expert.

Strand 6: LET EVERYTHING BE OKAY

As long as you pay proper attention and let things be okay, even mistakes can offer valuable learning opportunities. Better to instil good habits for a lifetime than be put off by an insignificant, short-term weight gain. To help with this, I recommend you do not weigh yourself for at least sixty days.

MAGIC ACTION STEP: Allow yourself to make mistakes.
MAGIC ACTION STEP: Give yourself permission to put on a little weight.

Strand 7: THE COMMITMENT TO HEROISM

This plan works only if you do it! This will require effort in the beginning, and there will be a temptation to give up. Remember, small steps outside your comfort zone create *huge* transformation.

If you would like faster weight loss, try intermittent fasting.

THAT'S IT! NOW, SET FORTH, AND BECOME THE HERO OF YOUR OWN LIFE!

WHERE TO GO FROM HERE

The Academy of Magic is a complete online magical membership. Students enjoy spellbinding teachings, a fabulous community and the chance to work more closely with Genevieve.
http://www.becomingmagic.com/academy-of-magic

For *Feasting on Magic* free resources
http://www.becomingmagic.com/feasting-resources

You can also complete the Magic Words 5 – Day Challenge. This is a free course I created to accompany or replace reading *Magic Words and How to Use Them*. Just visit this link to find out more
http://www.becomingmagic.com/magicwordscourse

If you'd like to find out more about how magic can help you, do visit Genevieve's website
http://www.becomingmagic.com